Visual Space Perception

Visual Space Perception

A Primer

Maurice Hershenson

A Bradford Book
The MIT Press
Cambridge, Massachusetts
London, England

This book was set in Bembo by Wellington Graphics and was printed and bound in the United States of America.

Library of Congress Cataloging-in-Publication Data

Hershenson, Maurice.
  Visual space perception : a primer / Maurice Hershenson.
    p.   cm.
  "A Bradford book."
  Includes bibliographical references and index.
  ISBN 0-262-08270-5 (hardcover : alk. paper). — ISBN 0-262-58167-1 (pbk. : alk. paper)
  1. Space perception. 2. Visual perception. I. Title.
  BF469.H45   1998 9
  152.141302   dc21

For Amy, who brings love and joy into every moment

Contents in Brief

Contents in Detail

Preface

Discussions of visual space perception usually take one of two forms—the obligatory recitation of "cues" found in undergraduate textbooks or the detailed description of specific topics found in handbooks. The former are relatively superficial and the latter so specific that neither provides students or scholars with a coherent overview. This book attempts to strike a balance between the two extremes. It presents a survey of the scientific study of visual space perception at a level that is, I hope, accessible to the undergraduate student while containing enough detail to be a source of basic knowledge for the scholar.

There is an important role for such a book. The renewed interest in the study of vision has attracted scholars from such diverse fields as artificial intelligence, engineering, mathematics, physics, neuroscience, and linguistics so that a single primer could provide a basis for additional study for scholars whose advanced training is in other fields. Furthermore, the development of virtual imaging devices and the popularization of stereoscopic effects in movies and posters has increased the interest level of beginning students. Both groups require more depth than is available in undergraduate texts and more breadth, in a manageable size, than is available in handbooks.

There are, of course, pitfalls in attempting to attain this goal. Topics must be selected that will present a representative overview and, within topics, specific theoretical positions and experimental findings must be selected to represent alternative conceptual positions and clearly established empirical findings. In some cases, these selections are clear but, in others, a judicious decision must be made.

There is no simple way to make such decisions. In general, they were guided by three questions: Does the phenomenon represent a basic process of the visual system? Are the data supporting the phenomenon or theory well established? Should students (undergraduates and scholars alike) know about this phenomenon in order to understand visual space perception? These questions are not easily answered because an observation that represents a basic process for one theoretical viewpoint may be an artifact for another. Therefore, in many cases, experimental observations are described in a theoretical context. Nevertheless, the topics discussed and the experiments described in this book represent one view of the basics of the field—the information that must be digested before one can begin to study visual space perception seriously.

There are two additional limitations that must be acknowledged. First, topics normally described as aspects of the study of sensation (e.g., color vision, masking) are not included. Second, brain anatomy and physiology are not described or discussed in detail. A few studies are mentioned to support the evidence but, in general, the data included come from psychophysical (behavioral) experiments.

The book has been greatly improved by the editorial comments of Robert P. O'Shea and an anonymous reviewer. Their hard work improved the accuracy, breadth, and clarity of the book and I thank them for it. However, I take full responsibility for any remaining errors.

The study of the aspect of consciousness we call visual space perception has provided me with countless hours of pleasure. If this book introduces others to the wonder and joy of seriously studying this remarkable achievement of our brains, I would feel it has been a worthwhile endeavor.

Visual Space Perception

The Problem of Visual Space Perception

The study of visual space perception begins with the assumptions that the physical world exists and that its existence is independent of the observer. The consequences of these assumptions are illustrated in figure 1.1. It shows a person looking at a scene containing the sky and the ground, as well as specific objects such as a house and a tree. It is not possible to observe the viewer's perception of this scene. Nevertheless, the viewer can describe the perception using two types of observable responses: verbal responses and motor responses. A verbal description of perception occurs when the viewer says, "I see a house over there." A motor response occurs when the viewer points at the house. Overt (observable) behaviors such as these are used to make inferences about the existence and properties of the viewer's perception, or the experience of seeing the house at a particular position in space.

The Physical World and the Perceptual World

The physical world exists outside the observer. The *perceptual* or *visual world* is experienced by the observer. It is produced by activity in the eye-brain system when patterned light stimulates the eyes of an observer. The perceptual world consists of the ground and the sky, as well as objects (including people) that are in view at a given moment. The perceptual world is normally *externalized*, i.e., it is usually experienced as "out there." (Visual sensations can be experienced internally by striking the eyeball or by stimulating the brain with electrical current. They sometimes occur in dreams or hallucinations.)

The perceptual world is experienced as a world containing objects that move about in a three-dimensional (3D) space. Most observers are aware of the volume of space as a quality of their experience. They are frequently less aware of the fact that their experience is taking place over time, although

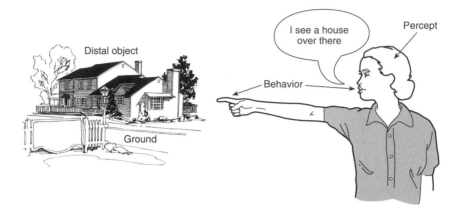

Figure 1.1
A person looking at a house and a tree on the ground, with the sky beyond. The
viewer's perception of the scene cannot be observed by another person. However,
the verbal and motor responses can be observed. This viewer reports seeing the
house at a particular place (verbal response) and points toward the house (motor
response).

the passage of time can easily be noticed when pointed out. Thus, the
perceived world is a four-dimensional world—3D space plus time.

The perceived world of the ground and sky is the space within which
we as observers exist. We move about in this space and interact with objects
in it. This space has attributes such as depth, distance, location, direction,
and motion, all of which can vary. Objects in this space have qualitative,
intensive, and spatial attributes such as size (extension), shape, constancy
(stability and rigidity), motion or movement, direction, and position (distance). Thus, perceived space is a four-dimensional world of objects with
attributes—a perceived 3D world filled with objects, some of whose attributes change over time.

Geometrical Relationships

Both the physical world and the perceptual world have structure. The
structure of these worlds and the relationships between the structures can
be described by geometry.

Physical Space

In the study of visual space perception, it is generally assumed that physical
space can be described by Euclidean geometry. In this space, an object can

be displaced or rotated without deformation, i.e., without changes between related points. The basis of Euclidean geometry is the *parallel postulate,* which states that parallel lines do not meet. For the purpose of studying perception, it is assumed that Euclidean geometry provides a good approximation of the structure of the physical world. Consequently, points in space can be assigned coordinates in a Cartesian (rectangular) coordinate system, and distances between points can be measured in units along three orthogonal axes (x, y, and z axes) that intersect at an origin. Two additional assumptions describe the physics of light: (1) light travels in straight lines and (2) when light is reflected from a surface, the angle of reflection is equal to the angle of incidence.

Perceptual (Visual) Space

The geometry of visual space is unknown and, therefore, must be determined empirically. This geometry must be different from that of physical space because it must take the perceiver into account. When visual space is described with respect to the perceiver, at least two qualities of perceived space can be distinguished: direction and distance. Note that these qualities of space only have meaning when there is a referent—the perceiver. Therefore, direction and distance from a perceiver are usually described using polar coordinates. A polar coordinate system refers the perceived qualities to a single point, a single real eye or the center of the "body image" (e.g., the bridge of the nose) of the viewer. By specifying an origin that corresponds to a perceiver, it is possible to measure visual space in terms of angular direction and radial distance from the origin.

Relationships among Spaces

The analysis of relationships between perceived and physical spaces must describe in precise terms the important characteristics of the physical objects and spaces, the patterns of stimulation they produce on receptor surfaces, and the perceptions resulting from this stimulation. The first relationship is between physical objects or scenes and the pattern of reflected light impinging on the retinal surfaces. To maintain the important distinction between these two aspects of stimulation, physical objects and scenes are described as *distal* stimuli and impinging patterns of light are described as *proximal* stimuli. (The use of the terms proximal and distal to describe stimuli should not be confused with their usage in anatomy or physiology describing parts of the body.) *Perception* refers to the process or act of perceiving, whose content is the *percept,* the conscious experience of the distal object or scene.

Distal objects and scenes can be observed directly. Proximal stimulus patterns can be observed by projecting light from distal stimuli onto a surface, a screen or projection plane that represents the retinal surface. Perception cannot be observed directly. Therefore, in the scientific study of perception, an additional component must be included in every observation of an act of perceiving—there must be an observable behavioral response to indicate that a particular perception is occurring. Thus, in experimental situations, instructions or training are used to produce behavioral responses that can be observed by an experimenter.

Each component of the perceptual act—distal stimulus, proximal stimulus, percept, response—can be described geometrically. Consequently, the relationship between adjacent components in the sequence may be described by mapping the geometry of one component into the geometry of the next component. For example, the Euclidean geometry of the 3D distal world can be mapped into its representation in the proximal stimulus on the two-dimensional (2D) receptor surface, and the proximal stimulus can be mapped into the 3D world of perception centered on the perceiver.

In the analysis of perception, the mapping of one geometry into another can be confusing because the same term may be used to describe qualities in both systems. For example, the term *size* may represent an attribute of a distal object as well as an attribute of a perceived object. Thus, the edge of a distal object may be a particular physical size but it may appear (in perception) to be a different size. To avoid confusing properties that have similar names in the physical and perceptual domains, the following conventions are adopted in this book: In the text, qualifiers such as *distal* and *proximal* are used whenever there is a possibility of confusion. In equations, physical (distal) quantities are described using upper-case letters and psychological (perceived) quantities are described using lower-case letters.

Distal–Proximal Relationships

ProjectIve Geometry: Geometrical Optics

The light falling on an eye can come directly from an emitting source. More frequently, however, it is light reflected from the surfaces of the ground and from objects on the ground. Light may also reach the eye after being

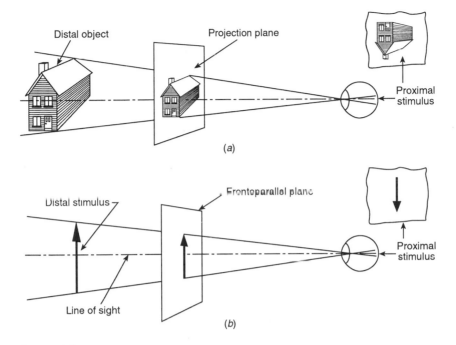

Figure 1.2
(a) Distal-proximal relationships for a viewer looking at a house. Light reflected from the house, a distal object, converges toward the eye and stimulates the retina. The image is inverted in the proximal stimulus. This pattern can be observed right-side up by projecting onto a frontoparallel plane between the viewer and the distal object. (b) Distal-proximal relationships for a single contour.

refracted through a medium such as air or water. The 2D pattern of light reflected to an eye from the 3D arrangement of objects in the world is described by *projective geometry*. Because this geometrical analysis is applied to light, it is called *geometrical optics*.

Light rays are reflected in all directions from a given point on a distal surface. However, in the study of perception, it is necessary to consider only the rays that enter the eye of a viewer. The collection of such rays can be indicated by their envelope, the two outer rays of any given bundle of rays. To simplify the geometrical optics relating distal to proximal stimuli, it can be assumed that light rays entering the eye cross at a single point. This point, the *nodal point* of the eye, or *optic node,* represents the optical properties of the eye and corresponds roughly to the center of rotation of the eye.

Figure 1.2 shows the distal-proximal relations for a single eye. In figure 1.2a, the viewer is looking at a house, a distal object. Light is reflected in every direction from every point on the house (excluding the windows). However, the perceiver is stimulated only by the light that enters the eye. This light is represented by the rays that converge toward the nodal point of the eye and stimulate cells on the retina of the viewer. The pattern of light stimulating the retina constitutes the *proximal stimulus*. The proximal image is inverted with respect to the orientation of the distal object. The proximal pattern can be observed right-side up by projecting onto a fronto-parallel plane between the viewer and the distal object.

Proximal Geometry: Geometry of Perspective

The structure or pattern of the proximal geometry can be represented in a hypothetical projection plane erected between the viewer and the distal stimulus. Figure 1.2b is a simplified representation of these relationships. In this diagram, the projection is on a *frontoparallel plane* or *picture plane,* a plane that is perpendicular to the line of sight of the viewer. The upright pattern in the proximal stimulus is described by the 2D geometry of perspective (see chapter 7 for details). In this pattern, the size of a distal object is represented according to the distance of the plane from the viewer.

The Problem of Visual Space Perception

The problem for the student of visual space perception is to relate the experienced qualities of visual space to specific aspects of stimulation and to processes occurring in the visual system. To simplify the task of identifying these components, it is necessary to divide the field of visual space perception in two different ways. First, it can be separated into perception with one eye (monocular perception) or two eyes (binocular perception). Second, it can be divided into static and kinetic analyses, depending on whether the proximal stimulus is changing or not. Binocular perception is discussed first (chapters 2 to 5) because the problems of perception are more easily demonstrated for two-eyed vision and because the processes have been worked out in more detail. For the same reason, static stimulation is discussed before kinetic stimulation.

I

Binocular Perception

The discussion of visual space perception begins with binocular perception. Chapter 2 explains visual directions, the arrangement of perceived points in space, up-down and left-right, with respect to the straight ahead. Chapter 3 begins the discussion of stereoscopic (binocular) depth perception. It explains the concepts of retinal disparity, fusion, and the horopter. Chapter 4 describes depth perception produced by traditional stereograms containing contour disparity. Chapter 5 describes cyclopean depth perception, stereoscopic depth perception produced by random-dot stereograms, and autostereograms.

2

Spatial Localization: Visual Directions

Different parts of the physical world appear to be in different directions—straight ahead, left or right, up or down. The study of visual direction is the study of our perceptions of the direction of objects in space, or the perceived frontal plane position of a stimulus with respect to the observer. Monocular visual directions can be related to the anatomical and optical properties of a single eye. Visual directions experienced when viewing a scene with two eyes are more complicated because the eyes are in different positions in space. Consequently, when looking at a single distal point, the two eyes must be oriented in slightly different directions. The discussion begins with a description of the monocular and binocular visual fields, the portions of the world that are visible to a stationary viewer.

Monocular Localization of Directions

The retina is the complex layered structure at the back of the eyeball that contains light-sensitive cells. The most sensitive area of the retina is near its center, the *yellow spot* or *macula lutea,* about 4 deg in diameter (see the appendix for a description of angular measurements). The center of this region contains the foveal pit. The *fovea,* the area across the top of the foveal pit, measures about 2 deg in diameter. The *foveola,* the area at the bottom of the pit, measures about 0.5 deg in diameter. When the eye fixates a distal point, the light from that point falls on the center of the foveola. At a given instant, with fixation on a single point, only a portion of the physical world is visible. The portion of the world that is visible to a single stationary eye defines the monocular visual field.

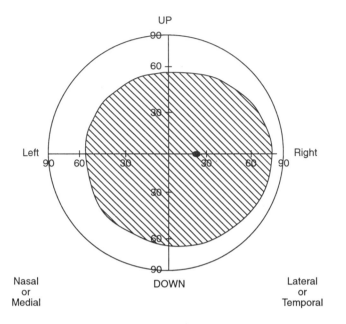

Figure 2.1
The monocular field of vision of the right eye projected onto a frontal plane. The blind spot is 15 to 16 deg to the nasal side of the fovea and projects to the temporal side of the field of vision.

Monocular Visual Field

The *monocular visual field* maps the extent of vision in all directions for a single stationary eye. To plot the monocular field, imagine a plane perpendicular to the line of sight of the eye, a *frontoparallel* or *frontal plane*. The viewer fixates a point in the plane with one eye. A second point in the plane is moved away from the first point toward the periphery until it is no longer visible. The position of the point when it is last visible marks the extent of the monocular field in that direction. The visual field may also be mapped by moving a point that is not visible toward the center of the field until it just becomes visible. This procedure, known as *perimetry,* is repeated in all directions around the point of fixation to map out the field.

Figure 2.1 shows a monocular field for the right eye for a bright stimulus. The field is not symmetrical because facial features such as the nose and the bony ridge above the eye block vision in some directions. The field extends approximately 60 deg up and 75 deg down; 100 deg to the right (lateral or temporal direction) and 60 deg to the left (medial or nasal direction), depending on individual facial characteristics (Henson, 1993).

Figure 2.2
Demonstration of the blind spot. Hold the book about 12 inches from the eyes.
Close your right eye and fixate the star with the left eye. Move the book slowly
toward or away from you until the disc is no longer visible.

The field is also affected by a number of other factors such as the intensity
of light and the type of stimulus used.

A small area on the retinal surface contains no receptor cells because
that is where the optic nerve leaves the eye. This area (15 to 16 deg to the
nasal side of the center) is called the *optic disc* or *blind spot*. Normally, the
blind spot is not seen. However, we can be made aware of it by closing one
eye, fixating a point with the other eye, and moving a second point into the
area of the field that corresponds to the blind spot. The second stimulus point
will not be visible. This procedure can easily be performed using figure 2.2.

Binocular Visual Field
If the monocular fields for the two eyes are superimposed, the portion of
the distal world that stimulates both eyes can be determined. This area is
the *binocular visual field* illustrated in figure 2.3. All distal points that stimulate
areas within the binocular visual field stimulate both eyes. Stimulation
within the binocular visual field is responsible for binocular depth perception or stereopsis (chapters 3 through 5). With both eyes open, the maximum width of the visual field is approximately 200 deg depending on the
projection of the nose. The binocular field is approximately 120 deg wide,
i.e., 60 deg on either side of the vertical midline. It is flanked by two
uniocular fields (the monocular temporal crescents), approximately 40 deg
wide (Henson, 1993). The vertical dimensions are the same as those of the
monocular fields. Note that the blind spots are covered uniocularly.

Objective Directions: Visual Lines
A *visual line* is the locus of distal points that stimulate a given point on the
retina of a single eye. The *principal visual line (PVL)* is the locus of distal
points that stimulate the center of the foveola of a single eye. This line
passing through the center of the foveola, the nodal point of the eye, and

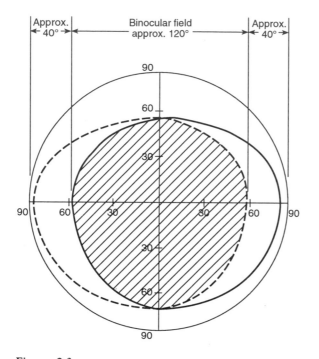

Figure 2.3
The binocular field of vision projected onto a frontal plane. The binocular field is surrounded by two uniocular fields, the monocular temporal crescents.

the fixated point, is the *visual axis* of the eye. It is different from the *optic axis,* which passes through the centers of the cornea and lens surfaces but not the center of the fovea.

Figure 2.4 shows the relationship between distal points and their representation in the proximal stimulus for a single eye. The lower portion of the figure shows a perspective view of these relations, looking at the retina from behind. The eye is shown fixating point P. Light from the fixated point falls on the center of the foveola *(P_r)*. The visual line connecting P with its retinal image point is the principal visual line, the visual axis of the eye. Point A is in the upper left quadrant of the distal field at a horizontal distance x and a vertical distance y from P. Light from his point stimulates the eye in the lower right quadrant *(A_r)*, displaced by an amount x_r in the horizontal direction and y_r in the vertical direction.

Subjective Directions: Visual Directions
Perceived *visual directions* are the subjective directions of points in space (up, down, left, right). When the eye is directed at a given point, the image of

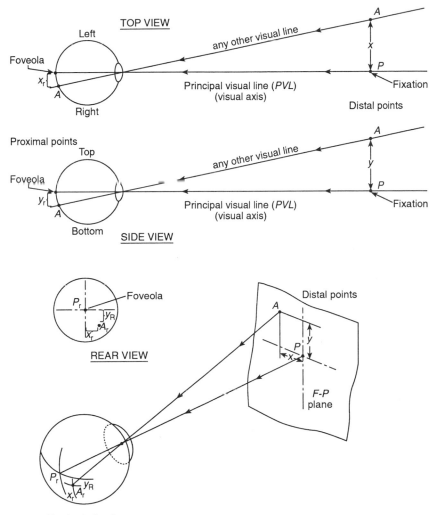

Figure 2.4
Distal-proximal relations described by visual lines. The eye is directed at point P. The visual axis (principal visual line) passes through this point, the nodal point of the eye, and the center of the foveola. Another point (A), x units to the left and y units up from P, projects to the lower right quadrant of the retinal surface.

that point falls on the center of the fovea. The subjective direction associated with this fixation is called the *principal visual direction (pvd)*. Each point in the retinal mosaic gives rise to a subjective visual direction which is described relative to the principal visual direction (the fixated direction). Figure 2.5 shows the relationships between proximal points and their perceived directions. Point A_r in the proximal stimulus appears to be in a direction that can be described by its vertical and horizontal angular displacement—it appears β deg to the left and θ deg up from the straight-ahead.

In the nineteenth century, Lotze (Pastore, 1971) proposed that the retina represents a mosaic of light-sensitive elements that, together with the processing activity they initiate, act as functional *local signs*. He recognized, moreover, that stimulation of specific receptors is not in itself sufficient to account for the perception of visual direction. There must also be a mechanism that analyzes the position of the stimulated receptors, the local signs, relative to the body as the center (origin) of the subjective directional coordinate system.

Vergence Movements

Binocular fixation on an object means that each eye is positioned so that the image of the object falls at the center of the foveola, the region that provides the most accurate vision (Alpern, 1962). With fixation on a distal point, the lines of sight (the visual lines through the point and the centers of rotation of each eye) intersect at that point forming an angle, the *convergence* or *apex angle*.

Eye movements are classified according to their effect on the convergence angle. *Version* movements are conjunctive eye movements that maintain a constant convergence angle, i.e., the eye muscles move the two eyes equally to the left or right, up or down. *Vergence* movements are disjunctive eye movements in which the convergence angle changes, i.e., the eye muscles move the eyes equally inward or outward. *Convergence* is movement toward the center line and *divergence* is movement away from the center line. In general, version movements are abrupt shifts and vergence movements are gradual changes. In binocular vision, vergence movements permit fixation on a point. *Fusional vergence* movements of the eyes bring the images of an object onto the foveas of the two eyes, the areas of highest visual acuity, resulting in a single fused image in perception.

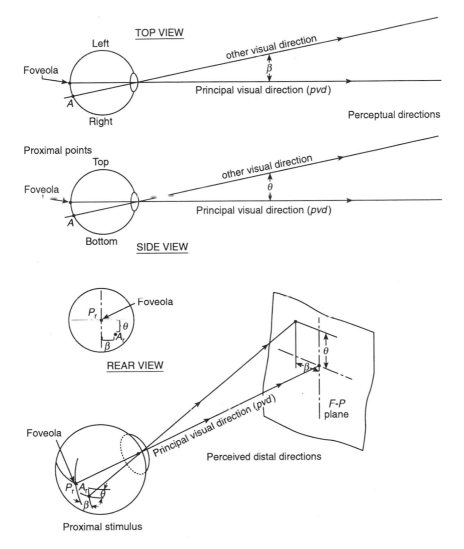

Figure 2.5
Proximal–perceptual relations described by visual directions. Perceived directions are described relative to the principal visual direction *(pvd)*. Point *A* appears to be β deg to the left and θ deg above the *pvd*.

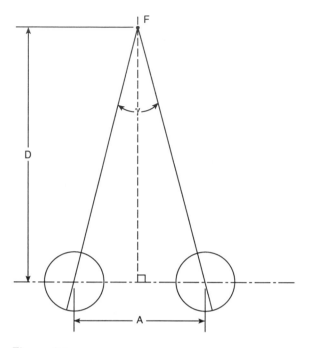

Figure 2.6
The convergence angle with symmetrical convergence: γ = convergence angle; *A* = interpupillary distance or distance between centers of rotation of the eyes; *D* = distance to fixation point *(F)* along the perpendicular bisector of *A*, i.e., in the median plane perpendicular to *A*.

Figure 2.6 illustrates symmetrical convergence produced by fixation on a point in the median plane, a plane perpendicular to the interocular axis. In general, the convergence angle or apex angle γ is given by:

$$\tan \gamma/2 = A/2D, \tag{2.1}$$

where *A* is the interpupillary distance, the distance between the centers of rotation of the two eyes, and *D* is the distance to a fixation point, *F*, in the median plane. For small angles (less than about 10 deg, where tan γ = γ in radians) equation 2.1 reduces to

$$\gamma = A/D \tag{2.2}$$

in radians, and

$$\gamma = (57.3)A/D \tag{2.3}$$

in degrees.

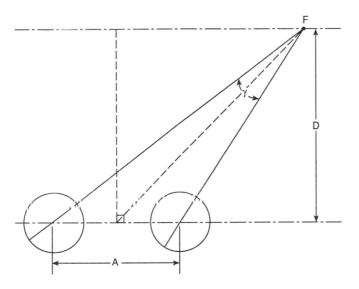

Figure 2.7
Convergence angle with asymmetrical convergence.

Figure 2.7 illustrates asymmetrical convergence produced by fixation on a point off the median plane. To a reasonable approximation, equation 2.3 also holds for this case (Graham, 1951).

Binocular Localization

The basic phenomena of binocular visual directions were demonstrated two centuries ago by Wells (1792/Ono, 1981, 1991).

Wells's Experiments
Figure 2.8 illustrates one simple experiment described by Wells. A rectangular piece of cardboard contains two lines forming a triangle with one of the edges. The line on the left is red and the line on the right is green. At the base of the triangle, the lines are separated by 2 to 3 inches (5 to 7.6 cm), the approximate distance between the eyes. The card is held just below eye level, with the bridge of the nose centered on the base of the triangle. With fixation on the apex of the triangle, a single line is seen extending from the nose to the fixation point. Parts of the line appear red and parts appear green, with the colors and positions changing over time. Two additional lines can be seen off to the sides directed toward the ears, a red line on the

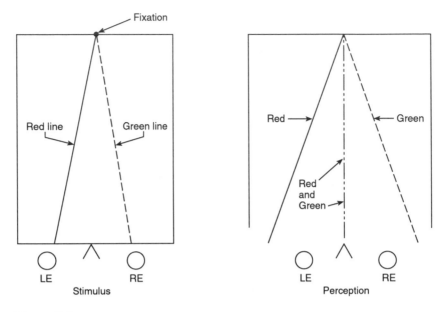

Figure 2.8
Wells's (1792/Ono, 1981) demonstration of binocular visual directions. The red and green lines approximate the *PVLs* to the left and right eyes, respectively. This stimulus is perceived as a single line, partly red and partly green, extending from the bridge of the nose to the fixation point.

left and a green line on the right. Monocular views can be compared with the binocular view by alternately opening and closing the eyes.

Figure 2.9 demonstrates the perception when the stimulus contains a single line running from the bridge of the nose to the fixation point. When viewed in this way, this line appears to be two lines going from the fixation point to each eye, respectively. Once again, alternately opening and closing the eyes can produce the respective monocular views.

Wells offered three propositions to explain the perception of binocular directions (Wells, 1792/Ono, 1981). Figure 2.10 demonstrates the propositions using Wells's "magic window" experiment. The stimulus consists of a card with two circular holes separated horizontally. The card is held in a frontal plane and a stimulus object is viewed through the holes in such a way that the left eye looks through the left hole and the right eye looks through the right hole. The viewer sees the fixated object directly in front of the nose through a "hole" in the cardboard. This outcome illustrates Wells's first proposition: that objects on the visual axes of the eyes (the holes)

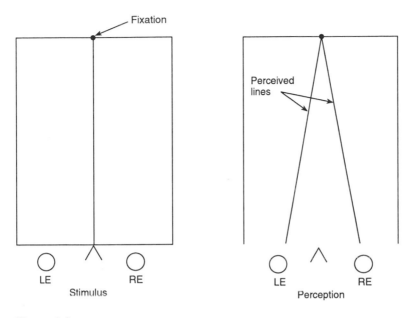

Figure 2.9
A stimulus consisting of a single line from the fixation point to the bridge of the nose appears to be two lines diverging from the fixation point, one to each eye (Wells, 1792/Ono, 1981).

are seen on a common axis, the line from the middle of the visual base (the space between the eyes) to the point of intersection of the axes.

The square between the holes in the stimulus card is seen as two squares, one on either side of the center hole. This outcome illustrates Wells's second proposition, which states that objects on the common axis (the square) appear on the visual axis of the nonviewing eye. This proposition can be understood by analyzing one eye at a time. The left eye views the fixation point through the left hole. The object on the common line (the square) is to the right of the left hole by an amount equal to the distance from the left hole to the center line. Therefore, when the hole is seen as straight ahead, the square is seen to the right of the perceived straight-ahead hole, on the visual line to the right eye. The reverse is true for the right eye and, when viewed binocularly, two squares are seen on the two visual axes.

Two additional holes are visible, one on either side of the two squares. This outcome can also be understood by analyzing one eye at a time. The left eye views the fixation point through the left hole, the square, and the

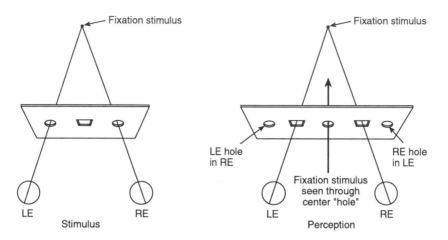

Figure 2.10
Wells's (1792/Ono, 1981) "magic window" experiment demonstrates all aspects of visual-direction phenomena (see text for details).

hole for the right eye view. With binocular vision, the left eyehole is seen as straight ahead, the square is seen to the right of the perceived straight-ahead hole (on the visual line to the right eye), and the right eyehole is seen to the right of the square. The reverse is true for the right eye. This outcome illustrates Wells's third proposition, which summarizes these complex relationships.

Cyclopean Eye

The conclusion of Wells's experiments is that, when looking with two eyes, we see the world as if from a single point. This is cyclopean vision and the point is described as the *cyclopean eye*. (*Cyclops* was a one-eyed monster in mythology.) Every perceived visual point has a single perceived visual direction from this cyclopean eye so that perceived directions are arranged egocentrically, straight ahead, up or down, to the right or to the left. Thus, binocular localization of visual directions is integrated and referred to a point which represents the felt position of the body, or *body image*. That is, the perceived direction of a point is determined by the locations of the images of the point on the two retinas and the positions of the eyes (usually determined by the fixation point).

The relationships between distal points, their proximal stimulus patterns, and their perceived directions are illustrated in figure 2.11. The eyes fixate point *F,* producing two principal visual directions, one for each eye.

This pattern of stimulation gives rise to a single perceived direction from a point approximately midway between the eyes d_F, the *primary subjective visual direction (psvd)*. Other points, such as *A* and *B*, also stimulate the two eyes. Their subjective directions *(d_A and d_B)* appear to emanate from the same point between the eyes. Thus, in general, directions are perceived as if arranged in a bundle, emanating from a point situated between the eyes, the cyclopean eye. Visual directions are sometimes called *egocentric directions* or *head-centric directions* because the reference system can be understood as centered about the viewer's head.

Note that there is not a one-to-one correspondence between the proximal stimulus (the retinal image) and perception. Two directions of stimulation give rise to a single direction in perception and, while two proximal points are stimulated, only one point is present in perception. Therefore the perceived direction is an *emergent* quality in perception, i.e., a quality in perception that is not in the proximal stimulus.

Law of Identical Visual Directions

Hering (1868/1977) called the relationships described above the *Law of Identical Visual Directions*: All objects lying in the paths of the chief rays to the foveas of the two eyes, i.e., on the two principal lines, will appear to be in the same primary subjective visual direction. For example, an object may be off to one side so that it is on a principal line to one eye and not to the other. Nevertheless, it will appear to be straight ahead, i.e., in the single primary subjective visual direction. This relationship holds over the entire visual field so that all points are seen relative to those that occupy the central portion of the retinas.

Hering's law can be observed by performing the simple experiment illustrated in figure 2.12. Look at a distant point through a window. Make two marks on the glass to correspond to the principal visual direction for each eye (best done with one eye at a time). These marks are separated laterally on the window but will be seen in the same visual direction when point *F* is viewed binocularly. The same is true with near fixation on a single point on the glass. Two far objects that are separated in space but fall on the principal lines of the two eyes, respectively, will appear to be in the same visual direction.

Hering's proposal that the cyclopean eye (the visual egocenter or center of projection) is located midway between the eyes has been challenged. A number of binocular situations have been found suggesting that localization

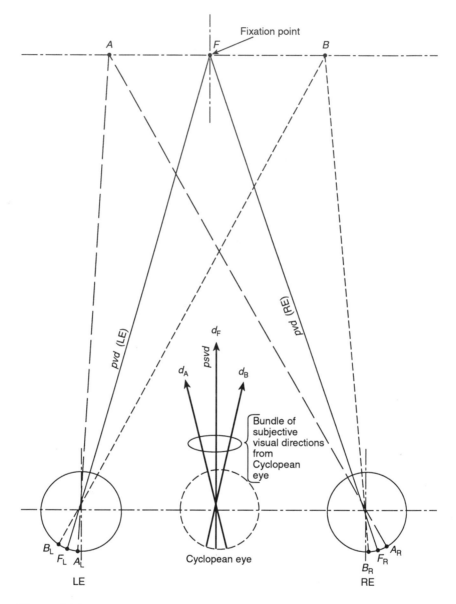

Figure 2.11
Cyclopean eye for visual directions summarizing the relationships between distal
points, proximal stimulus patterns, and perceived binocular directions.

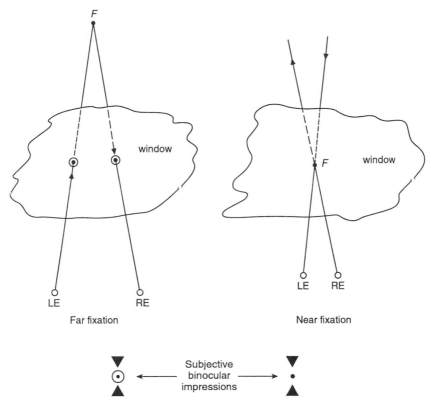

Figure 2.12
Demonstrations of Hering's Law of Identical Visual Directions (see text for details).

of the egocenter is biased toward the dominant eye and that information from the nondominant eye is suppressed or ignored (Porac & Coren, 1976, 1986). However, the data of Barbeito and Ono (1979; Barbeito, 1981; Ono & Barbeito, 1982) suggest that the center for visual directions is, indeed, located near the corneal plane midway between the eyes (see Ono, 1991, for a review).

Corresponding Points
If Hering's law is true, there must be a retinal element in one eye which, when stimulated, gives rise to the same subjective visual direction as an element in the other eye. In other words, the points are not seen in the actual directions of the stimulus to each eye—they appear to be in a single direction from the cyclopean eye. Points in the two eyes that demonstrate

such a relationship are said to be *corresponding points*. Thus, for a given fixation, every retinal point in the binocular field of one eye has a partner in the retina of the other eye with an identical directional value. Consequently, corresponding points may be defined as those points (one in each eye) that produce the perception of a single visual direction. Note that this is a functional definition, not an anatomical one, i.e., corresponding points refer to retinal points that function together in perception, not to retinal units that are physically connected (Ono, 1979, 1981, 1991).

Fusion

When a single distal point stimulates two eyes, two distinct retinal points are stimulated, one in each eye. Nevertheless, the point may be seen as a single point in space. This singleness of vision is described as *fusion*—the two proximal points have been "fused" into a single point in perception. Fusion is a second way to describe the perception produced by stimulation of corresponding points. There are also nonfixated corresponding points that are seen as single (fusion of noncorresponding points is discussed in chapter 3). Thus, when the two retinas are stimulated on corresponding points, the points are seen as single and localized in space at the intersection of the respective lines of direction from the two eyes.

Horopter and Vieth-Müller Circle

The "horizon of vision" or *horopter* is a concept introduced by Aguilonius in the seventeenth century to relate distal points to points in the two eyes according to the perceptual outcomes they produce (see Tyler, 1983, 1991b, for details). An early definition described the horopter as a distal surface that, for a given fixation, contains all the points whose images in the two eyes fall on corresponding retinal points. Consequently, each point on this horopter is seen as single and in a single visual direction (Gulick & Lawson, 1976; Ogle, 1962d). Modern research has shown, however, that different definitions and measurement procedures result in different forms of the horopter. Specifically, there is a longitudinal horopter, a point horopter, a fusion horopter, an equidistance horopter, and a frontoparallel plane horopter, each of which has a different form (Ogle, 1962d; Tyler, 1983, 1991b). The differences among the horopters are described in the next chapter.

The *Vieth-Müller circle* (V–M circle) is an early nineteenth–century attempt to find a simple geometrical relationship between distal points and

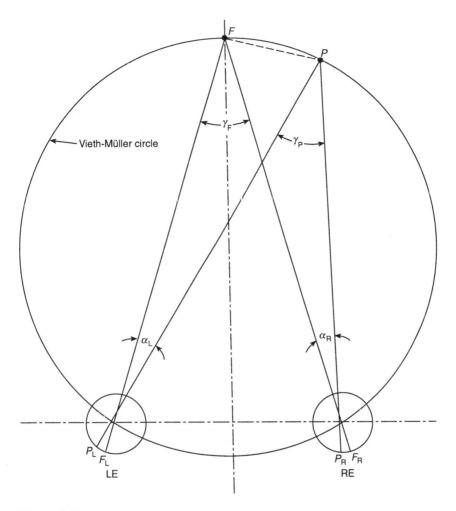

Figure 2.13
The Vieth–Müller circle passes through the fixation point and the centers of rotation
of the eyes. The convergence angles are equal for any pair of points on the V-M
circle $(\gamma_F = \gamma_P)$, and the angular separation of the points (visual angle) is the same
for both eyes $(\alpha_L = \alpha_R)$.

corresponding retinal points. It was based on the expectation that proximal points at the same lateral distance from the foveas of the two eyes would be corresponding points and, therefore, would subtend the same horizontal (longitudinal) angles. The resulting curve is a circle in a horizontal plane passing through the fixation point and the nodal points of the eyes.

The V-M circle is illustrated in figure 2.13. The eyes fixate point F, whose images, F_L and F_R, fall on the centers of the respective foveas. The images of point P, another point on the V-M circle, fall on P_L and P_R, respectively. All points on the circle subtend the same arc (defined by the separation between the eyes) and therefore have the same convergence angle, $\gamma_F = \gamma_P$. Furthermore, pairs of points on the circle are the same distance apart for each eye. Therefore, they subtend the same separation angle at the eyes, $\alpha_L = \alpha_R$.

Absolute Visual Directions

Visual directions have been described for a pair of stationary eyes, and perceived directions were related to the direction associated with a specific fixation. In real life, the observer is moving, and the head and eyes are also moving. Nevertheless, perceivers maintain a sense of their positions in space. They also maintain a sense of the *absolute visual directions* of objects, the spatial relations among objects in the environment that remain stable despite eye movements, changes in the fixation point, and perceiver motion. This absolute set of subjective directions permits orientation within the environment, i.e., the knowledge of one's own position and that of surrounding objects. This ability must take account of information in addition to the functional local signs of retinal points. It probably uses information in signals to the eye muscles to change fixation and to provide visual stimuli for a correction of the general sense of direction. When the directional system is influenced as a unit in this way, perceived space does not become deformed even though the retinal image is constantly changing. Only when this additional information is absent, as, for example, when the eye is moved by a finger, does the entire scene appear to move and deform (Ogle, 1962a).

Summary

The discussion of binocular vision began with the analysis of visual directions. A single distal point produces a proximal stimulus consisting of two points, one in each eye. Nevertheless, the observer experiences a single (fused) point in a single (cyclopean) direction. For a given fixation, the distal points that lie on a surface in space, the horopter, stimulate corresponding retinal points and result in fusion and perceived singleness of direction. The next chapter describes the perceptual consequences when noncorresponding retinal points are stimulated.

3

Stereopsis: Fusion and Horopters

Binocular depth perception or *stereopsis* may be thought of as a "sensation" (like seeing the color red), arising directly from stimulation of the two eyes when they are directed at the same point in space. Stereopsis contributes to perceived distance, the apparent distance of an object from the viewer, as well as to the perceived depth difference between objects or parts of objects. When the differences are among parts of the same object, stereopsis results in the perception of *solidity*. Stereopsis occurs over the entire binocular field. It produces accurate perceived relative depth up to about 135 meters (approximately 148 yards) and has been demonstrated in dim illumination, with rods as well as cones (Ogle, 1962b).

The Problem of Binocular Depth Perception

When a perceiver looks at an object, the stimulus patterns on the retinas of the two eyes differ because the eyes are located in different positions in space. These spatial relationships pose a problem for visual science because the object and the world around it appear unified, i.e., as a single object in a single world, despite the fact that the stimulus is represented differently on the receptor surfaces of the two eyes. This is the problem of *binocular parallax,* first described by Leonardo da Vinci (Boring, 1942).

Figure 3.1 illustrates Leonardo's paradox. It shows a schematic (top view) representation of a person looking at a cylindrical column in front of a wall. Sight lines delimit the portions of the column and back wall that reflect light to stimulate each eye. The sight lines from each eye are tangent to the circle that represents the column. The left eye is stimulated by light reflected from the cylindrical surface between A and C and by light reflected from the entire wall, except for that portion between A and C. The right

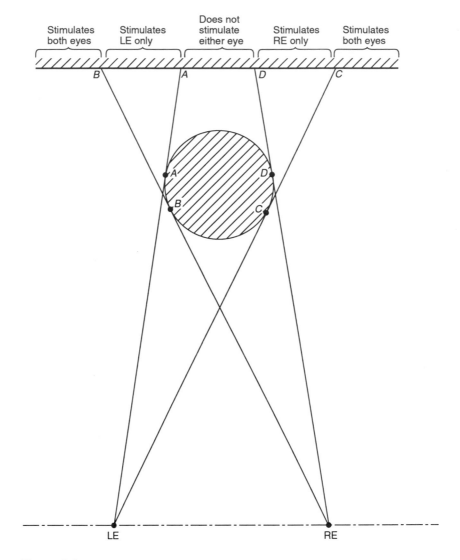

Figure 3.1.

Leonardo's paradox illustrates the problem of binocular vision. The eyes are in different positions in space and, therefore, are stimulated by different parts of the visual field. The figure shows the top view of a cylindrical column in front of a wall. The left eye is stimulated by light reflected from the column between points A and C and from the back wall except the portion between A and C. The right eye is stimulated by light reflected from the column between points B and D and from the back wall except the portion between B and D.

eye is stimulated by light reflected from the cylinder between *B* and *D* and from the back wall, except for the portion between *B* and *D*. The problem of binocular vision is to explain the perceptual system activity that permits us to see a single world of solid objects arrayed in depth, given these differences in the stimuli at the eyes.

Longitudinal Horopter and Retinal Disparity

The first step in solving the problem is to relate points in space to their retinal representations and to the perceptions they produce. The concept of the horopter serves this function. The *longitudinal horopter* is the most easily understood: It is the surface in space containing all points that, for a given fixation, stimulate corresponding retinal points in the two eyes. All points not on this surface (all other distal points) stimulate noncorresponding retinal points, resulting in a disparity between the two retinal images. The farther such points are from the horopter, the larger the *retinal disparity*. Horizontal retinal disparity is the necessary and sufficient condition for stereoscopic depth perception—the experience of a difference in depth (Wheatstone, 1838). Stereopsis appears to be a direct response to retinal disparity, and may not require interpretation or inference.

An alternative definition of the longitudinal horopter is that it is the locus of distal points that produce zero horizontal retinal disparity. It is known as the longitudinal horopter because it is equivalent to a horopter measured with long vertical lines, similar to the lines of longitude on a globe. This horopter is a 2D surface that has the form of a vertical cylinder passing through the V-M circle, with its center halfway between the eyes and the fixation point (Gulick & Lawson, 1976; Ogle, 1962d; Tyler, 1983, 1991b).

Figure 3.2 illustrates these relationships. Point *P* on the horopter surface projects to *P′* on a horizontal plane thorough *F,* the fixation point, and the centers of rotation of the eyes. All points on the vertical line (longitude) *P*-*P′* have the same horizontal separation from *F,* α_L in the left eye and α_R in the right eye. Therefore, any point on this line will stimulate corresponding points in the two eyes (Ogle, 1962d).

The relationships for the horizontal plane are illustrated in more detail in figure 3.3. The upper portion of the figure shows a top view of the eyes fixating a distal point, *F*. The lower portion of the figure illustrates the proximal stimulation in the two eyes when viewing the retinas from the rear. Point *F* is on the horopter and light reflected from that point falls on

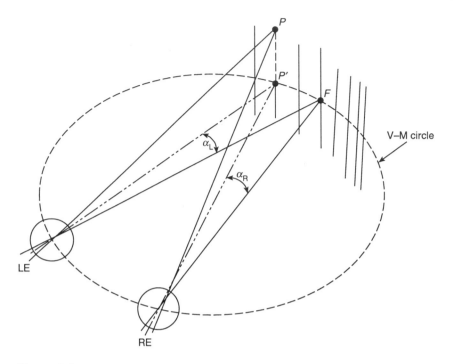

Figure 3.2
A perspective representation of the longitudinal horopter for fixation at F. Point P projects to P', a point in a horizontal plane through F (and on the V-M circle). Therefore, P and P' are at the same horizontal distance $(\alpha_L = \alpha_R)$ from F.

the centers of the two foveas, F_L and F_R. A second point, P, is also on the horopter. Light from P stimulates retinal points P_L and P_R on the horizontal axes of the eyes and to the left of center. Thus, the distal points F and P stimulate corresponding points F_L-F_R and P_L-P_R, respectively.

Figure 3.3 also shows two distal points that are not on the horopter: Point A is beyond the horopter and point B is closer than the horopter. To simplify the analysis, the points have been placed on the same visual line to the left eye as point P. Therefore, points A and B stimulate the left eye on the same point as point P. This is not the case for the right eye, however. Light from point A, the point beyond the horopter, falls on A_R, a retinal point that is more distant from the fovea than P_R. Light from point B, the point nearer than the horopter, falls on B_R, a retinal point nearer to the fovea than P_R. Thus, the images of points A and B do not fall on corresponding points in the two eyes.

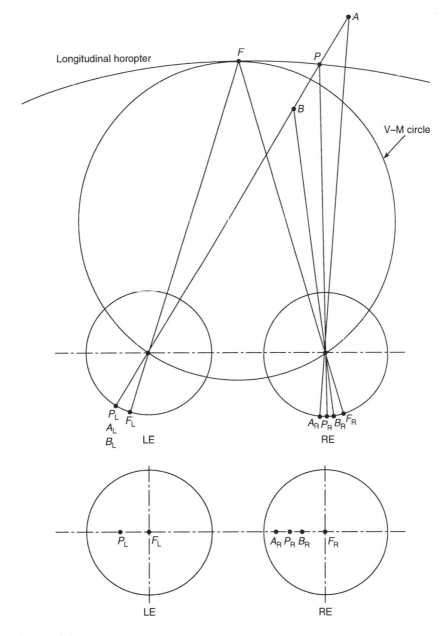

Figure 3.3
Relationships between distal points and proximal points for a person fixating distal point F. The lower diagram shows the proximal stimulus, viewing the retinas from the rear. Light from F falls on the centers of the two foveas, F_L and F_R. Light from a point P on the horopter stimulates retinal points P_L and P_R on the horizontal axes of the eyes, and to the left of center. Distal point A, beyond the horopter, and point B, closer than the horopter, stimulate the left eye on the same point as P. In the right eye, light from A falls on A_R, a retinal point that is more distant from the fovea than P_R, and light from B falls on B_R, a retinal point nearer to the fovea than P_R.

Retinal disparity is indexed by the difference in convergence angles (binocular parallax) between two points, with the farther point having a negative disparity relative to the nearer point. In figure 3.4, the eyes fixate point F at a distance, D_F, measured perpendicular to the interocular axis *(A)*. Another point P is at a distance, D_P. This point is off the horopter and closer to the viewer by δ, the difference between the distances of the two points: $\delta = D_F - D_P$. γ_F is the apex angle of the fixation point and γ_P is the apex angle of any other point P off the horopter. α_L is the angular separation of the two points in the left eye and α_R is the angular separation in the right eye. Retinal disparity is measured by the difference in the angles subtended in the two eyes by the lines of sight to the two points: $\alpha_L - \alpha_R$ This difference is equal to the difference in convergence angles with changed sign: $\alpha_L - \alpha_R = \gamma_P - \gamma_F$. Generally, the distance to the fixation point is very much larger than both A and δ ($D_F \gg A$ and δ) so that $\gamma_F = A/D$ and $\gamma_P = A/D \pm \delta$, in radians. Assuming $D \pm \delta$ is approximately equal to D, retinal disparity is given by:

$$\eta = Ad/D^2 \tag{3.1}$$

in radians. Cormack and Fox (1985) provide a detailed analysis of the simplifying assumptions on which this calculation of retinal disparity is based.

Fusion and Double Images

Retinal disparity produces different perceptual outcomes depending on the size and direction (crossed or uncrossed) of the disparity, among other things. To facilitate the description here, the outcomes from large disparities are described first so that directional differences can be illustrated in the perception of double images.

Double Images When Disparity Is Large
The disparity produced by noncorresponding points beyond the longitudinal horopter is opposite in direction to that produced by points closer than the horopter. The consequences of these directional differences in disparity can be observed when disparity is large and does not result in fusion. In this case, two distinct images of the points can be seen *(double images* or *diploplia)*. We are usually not aware of double images. However, if we attend to them,

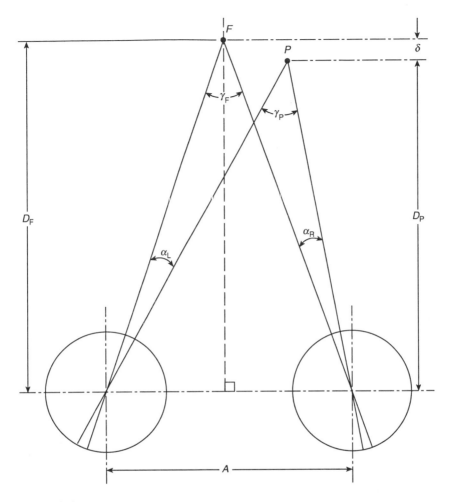

Figure 3.4
Calculation of retinal disparity η, where A = the interocular distance, F = the fixation point, P = a point off the horopter, D_F = the distance to F perpendicular to the interocular axis, D_P = the distance to P perpendicular to the interocular axis, δ = the difference in their distances (D_F - D_P), γ_F = the apex angle of the fixation point, γ_P = the apex angle of the other point, α_L = the visual angle separation of the points in the left eye, and α_R = the visual angle separation of the points in right eye.

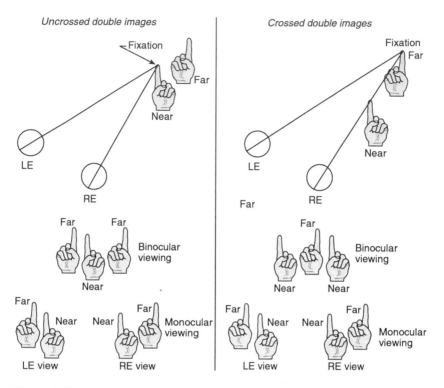

Figure 3.5

Demonstration of crossed and uncrossed double images. A point beyond the horopter (right index finger) will appear to the left of the fixation point (left index finger) in the left eye and to the right of the fixation point in the right eye. These are *uncrossed double images*. A point nearer than the horopter (left index finger) will appear to the right of the fixation point (right index finger) in the left eye and to the left of the fixation point in the right eye. These are *crossed double images*.

we see that the two images of a given distal point are in different visual directions for each eye.

The directional difference of double images can be observed using the procedure illustrated in figure 3.5. Fixate the tip of the left index finger placed about 12 inches (about 30 cm) in front of your nose. Align the right index finger about 6 inches (about 15 cm) behind it while maintaining fixation on the near finger. The finger behind the fixation point will appear double. Now alternately close your eyes. When you are looking with the left eye, the image of the far finger is to the left of the fixated finger and, when looking with the right eye, its image is to the right of the fixated finger. These images are described as *uncrossed double images*.

Now change fixation to the far finger and observe the double images of the near finger. Again, close your eyes alternately. This time, when seen with the left eye, the image of the near finger is to the right of the fixated finger and, when seen with the right eye, its image is to the left of the far finger. These images are described as *crossed double images*. The disparities produced by noncorresponding point stimuli are also described in terms of the positions of the points relative to the longitudinal horopter. Points more distant than the horopter produce *uncrossed disparities* and points nearer than the horopter produce *crossed disparities*.

Relative Depth and Fusion When Disparity Is Small

When the disparity is small, noncorresponding points appear single (fused) but at different distances from the viewer than points on the horopter. This relative depth difference is *stereoscopic depth perception*—depth perception from retinal disparity. Depending on the direction of the disparity, points appear either in front of or behind the longitudinal horopter surface. Uncrossed disparity in the proximal stimulus results in the perception of points behind the horopter and crossed disparity results in the perception of points in front of the horopter. The size of the fusional area around the horopter increases with eccentricity, i.e., with increasing horizontal distance from the fovea. It varies from a little less than 10 min in central vision to over 30 min near 15 deg in the periphery (Ogle, 1950/1964). Wheatstone (1838) first noted that the visual direction of a fused stimulus is a compromise between the directions seen from each eye *(allelotropia)*. Indeed, the visual direction of a point is the average of the visual directions predicted from the two monocular images (Ono, 1991; Sheedy & Fry, 1979).

Panum's Fusional Areas

When disparity is small, stimulation of disparate retinal points can result in fusion, the perception of a single point. Panum (1858; Tyler, 1983, 1991b) suggested that a stimulus in one eye could be fused with a similar stimulus in the other eye that fell on points near the point of precise correspondence. Thus, for a given pair of corresponding points, *Panum's fusional area* delimits the range of retinal disparities that result in a fused image. It can be represented as a small area surrounding corresponding points in the two eyes. In other words, when a distal point stimulates noncorresponding retinal points in the two eyes and these retinal points fall within Panum's area, the perceptual image is fused even though the retinal points are disparate.

These relationships are illustrated in figure 3.6 showing a fixation point, F, and a second point, P, on the horopter. The relative positions of these points on the retinas of the two eyes, looking from behind the head, are illustrated in the lower part of the figure. The fixation point stimulates the centers of the foveas of the two eyes, F_L and F_R, respectively. Point P stimulates corresponding points in the two eyes, P_L and P_R, respectively. Point A is far off the horopter between point P and the left eye, directly on the visual line from point P. It stimulates point A_L, the same point as P_L in the left eye. But the stimulus in the right eye is different. The point does not stimulate P_R because it is off the horopter. Instead, it stimulates A_R, a noncorresponding point. These retinal points have a large disparity between them and therefore result in the perception of double images, i.e., A_L and A_R do not fuse.

If P is seen as single and A is seen as double, somewhere between the positions of P and A there must be a transition from fusion to double images. This is the point marked B. This point stimulates the same point in the left eye as A and P. However, in the right eye, it stimulates B_R, a point between P_R and A_R. Stimulation of the right eye anywhere between B_R and P_R results in fusion. In addition, transition points similar to B must exist in all directions around P so that an area can be marked off in the right eye around P_R in such a way that stimulation anywhere in this area will fuse with stimulation of point P_L. This area is *Panum's area*. Figure 3.7 summarizes the relationships between fusion, double images, and the longitudinal horopter.

In its traditional conception, Panum's area was a fixed property of a given retinal region. It is now understood that this view is incorrect—the size and shape of Panum's area depends on the spatial and temporal characteristics of the stimulus as well as on the procedures used to measure it. For example, Tyler (1973) presented a straight line to one eye and a sinusoidal wavy line to the other eye. When the lines were horizontal (producing vertical disparity), the threshold for fusion remained relatively constant. However, when the lines were vertical (producing horizontal disparity), Panum's areas varied markedly with the size of the wave. The horizontal displacement varied from 2 to 60 min, a thirtyfold variation in fusion limits.

In another study of stimulus size, Schor, Wood, and Ogawa (1984) found that larger objects remained fused over a greater range of disparities than smaller objects, and that blurred images remained fused over a greater

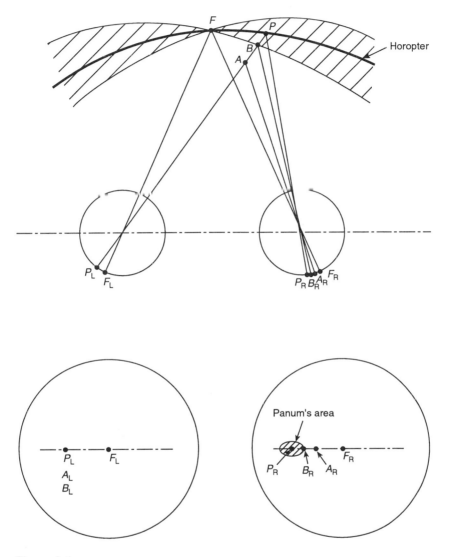

Figure 3.6

Panum's area. Point A is off the horopter on the visual line from P. It stimulates A_L in the left eye and a noncorresponding point, A_R, in the right eye. These retinal points have a large disparity and therefore result in the perception of double images. If A is moved toward P, fusion occurs at some point before reaching P. This point B stimulates B_R, a point between P_R and A_R. If point B is moved in all directions around P, an area in the right eye can be marked off around P_R in such a way that stimulation anywhere within this area will fuse with stimulation of point P_L.

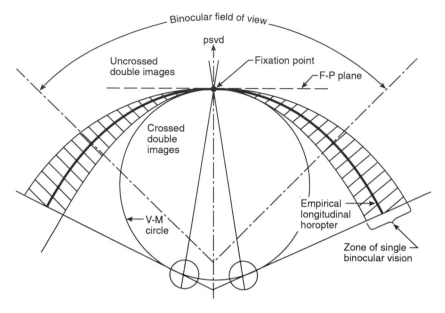

Figure 3.7
Summary of relations between zone of fusion, double images, and longitudinal horopter.

range than images that were sharply focused. Schor and Tyler (1981) varied spatial and temporal characteristics simultaneously. They found that the vertical dimensions of Panum's areas remained relatively constant whereas the horizontal dimensions varied from a maximum of 20 to a minimum of 1.5 min. At low temporal and spatial frequencies, Panum's areas were elliptical with a ratio of 2.5 to 1 between the horizontal and vertical axes and, at high temporal frequencies, the areas were circular. Schor, Heckmann, and Tyler (1989) found that the frequency content of the features of a stimulus determined the limits of fusion, whereas stimulus characteristics such as contrast and phase relations between spatial frequency components did not.

Disparate retinal images can cause the eyes to move so that the images fall as near as possible onto corresponding retinal elements. The consequences of these fusional movements is that the disparity is eliminated and the appearance of double images is prevented. Fusional movements can be initiated by retinal disparity in the peripheral as well as the central parts of the binocular visual field (Ogle, 1962c). An experimental demonstration of fusion compulsion is illustrated in figure 3.8. The eyes are fixated on point

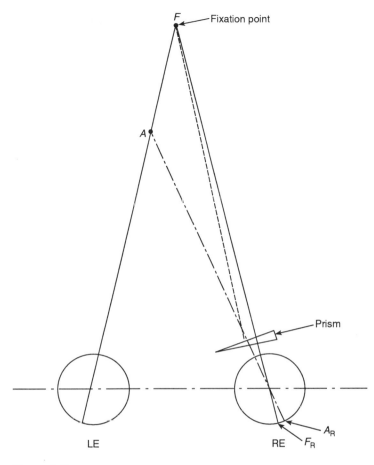

Figure 3.8
Demonstration of compulsion for fusion. When the prism is inserted, the light from F is refracted and stimulates A_R. In response, the right eye shifts toward A, resulting in the perception of a single fused point at A.

F and a prism is inserted between F and the right eye. The prism shifts the light falling on the retina of the right eye from F_r to A_r. The right eye then rotates so that it is directed at point A, resulting in the perception of a single point (fusion) at A.

Different Horopters

Although the classical literature frequently describes *the* horopter (usually meaning the longitudinal horopter), it has become clear that there is no single horopter. The shape and form of a horopter depends on its definition and on the procedures used to measure it (Tyler, 1991b).

Vertical and Torsional Disparity, Cyclofusion

The classical study of stereoscopic vision stressed horizontal retinal disparities. However, the visual system also produces fusional responses when stimulated by vertical and torsional (or orientational) disparities. Thus there is a component of the fusional response in each of the three orthogonal directions along which disparity can vary. Vertical disparities do not give rise to depth perception but they can degrade perceived depth from horizontal disparity (Ogle, 1962c; Tyler, 1983, 1991b). The response to torsional disparity is called *cyclofusion*. This term describes both the fused percept and the rotations of the eyes about the line of sight called *cyclovergent movements* (see Kertesz, 1991, for details).

Longitudinal Horopter, Point Horopter, and Fusion Horopter

The *point horopter* is the locus of distal points that result in zero retinal disparity, i.e., when both vertical and horizontal disparities are zero. It is different from the *longitudinal horopter,* which relates only to horizontal disparities (ignoring vertical disparities). The locus of points with zero vertical disparity, the *vertical horopter,* is a straight line in the vertical midline that passes through the fixation point and is tilted backwards in depth at the top, passing approximately through the feet at the bottom. Therefore, the point horopter is a line structure embedded in the cylindrical longitudinal horopter surface of horizontal disparity. Ideally, the point horopter is a horizontal circle (the V–M circle) and a vertical line intersecting at the fixation point. Its structure is a consequence of the geometry of binocular projection space which produces vertical disparities for object points off the V–M circle (Ogle, 1962c; Tyler, 1983, 1991b).

The *fusion horopter* is the locus of distal points that result in the perception of a single (fused) point. With discovery of Panum's fusional areas, this horopter could no longer be described as a surface. It had to have thickness—a dimension in depth—with the fusional area getting larger with increasing peripheral angle. The structure of this horopter, determined empirically, is a 3D volume around the line structure of the point horopter, i.e., a circle or conic section that is approximately horizontal and a vertical line that tilts back at the top by an amount that varies with fixation distance (Tyler, 1983, 1991b). The thickness of the fusional regions around these lines also varies with fixation distance. The fusion horopter expands and contracts according to the nature of the stimulus and the characteristics of the viewer's eyes. In other words, it is not a fixed property of vision—it is only an indication of the range of fusion (see Arditi, 1986; Tyler, 1991a, 1991b, for reviews).

Distance Horopters: Equidistance and Frontoparallel Plane Measurements

The *equidistance horopter* is the locus of points that appear to be at the same distance from the viewer. It is different from the binocular disparity horopter and has no geometric relation to it. An empirical measurement of this horopter is obtained by moving stimulus objects so they appear to be equidistant from the viewer. Theoretically, the equidistance horopter is a sphere centered on the observer's eyes and about double the diameter of the correspondence (longitudinal) horopter (Tyler, 1991b). The *frontoparallel plane horopter* is the locus of points that appear to be in the same frontal plane. An empirical measurement of this horopter is obtained by moving stimulus objects radially so they appear to form an apparent frontoparallel plane.

Hering-Hillebrand Deviation

Early measurements of the longitudinal horopter (Hering, 1864; Hillebrand, 1893) produced distance horopters between the V-M circle and the fronto-parallel plane through the fixation point. This deviation from the V-M circle is known as the *Hering-Hillebrand deviation*. Ogle's (1950/1964) measure-ments of this distance horopter are summarized in figure 3.9 with data from different graphs (note different dimensions). For fixation at 6 meters (about 20 feet), the horopter approximates a frontal plane; for fixation closer than 6 meters, the horopter curves toward the viewer (but is not a V-M circle); and for fixation farther away than 6 meters, the horopter curves away from the viewer. The degree of curvature becomes greater the further the fixation point is from 6 meters.

Thus, the geometry of perceived distances in visual space is not Euclid-ean. There are systematic differences between physical space and perceived binocular space. These differences have been measured by Foley (1966, 1967) using different tasks: Observers moved stimuli so that they appeared to lie in the same frontoparallel plane, or on the same equidistant circle as a fixed element; or bisected the distance between the viewer and a stimulus point. Foley found that, in each task, there was one distance at which the

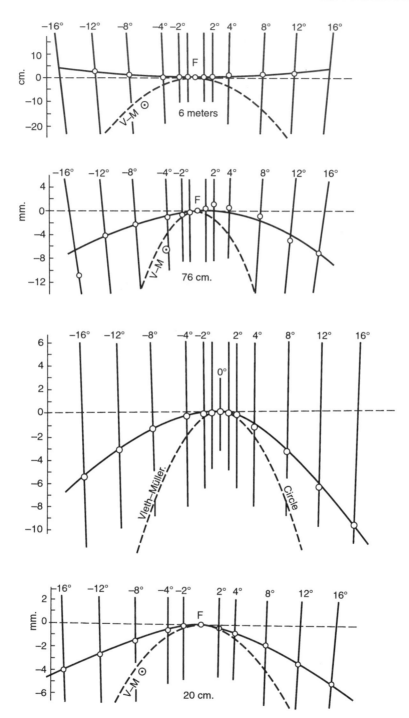

perceived array of points corresponded to the theoretical (physically correct) position of the points. This distance generally was between 1 and 4 meters. There were systematic errors at other distances: Points at nearer distances were set too close and points at farther distances were set too far (Foley, 1966, 1967, 1980, 1991).

Summary

This chapter described the relationships between points in space, their projections to points on the two retinas, and the perceptions associated with them. The longitudinal horopter is the locus of distal points that produce zero horizontal disparity. Points off the horopter produce horizontal retinal disparity resulting in stereoscopic depth perception. Small disparities produce the perception of a fused, single point. Large disparities produce diploplia, the perception of double images. Chapter 4 advances the study of stereopsis from points to solid objects with surfaces and edges.

Figure 3.9
The Hering-Hillebrand deviation from the V-M circle. Empirical measurements of the apparent frontoparallel plane horopter approximate a frontal plane at about 6 meters. Closer fixation produces a horopter that is curved toward the viewer, and fixation farther away produces a horopter that is curved away from the viewer. (By permission of Mayo Foundation. Figures 11 and 16 from Ogle, K. N., 1950/1964. *Researches in binocular vision.* New York: Hafner Publishing Co.)

4

Stereopsis: Traditional Stereograms

Stereoscopes are devices that permit slightly different stimulus patterns to be viewed dichoptically, i.e., one pattern with the left eye and a different pattern with the right eye. When the appropriate patterns are used, the viewer sees solid objects in 3D space. Charles Wheatstone constructed the first mirror stereoscope about 1833 and David Brewster constructed the first prism stereoscope about 1849 (see Gulick & Lawson, 1976, for a discussion of the history and controversy surrounding these discoveries).

Stimulus Components of Stereoscopic Half-Images

The stimuli presented to the respective eyes are stereoscopic half-images. For many years, stereoscopic depth perception was understood as a direct consequence of the retinal disparity of contours or edges in the half-images. There are, however, other differences in the half-images—the perspective representation and the occlusion patterns are slightly different because the eyes are in different positions in space.

Contour or Edge Disparity

In chapter 3, retinal disparity was described for points in space. However, the real world consists of solid objects, usually scattered around on the ground. Consequently, the early study of stereopsis was based on the analysis of 2D representations of the outline shapes of objects, and the early stereoscopes were based on retinal disparity produced by the contours or edges of these objects.

Figure 4.1 illustrates the patterns produced in each eye by the edges of a cube situated directly in front of a viewer. The upper portion of the figure shows the cube in perspective and the lower portion shows a top

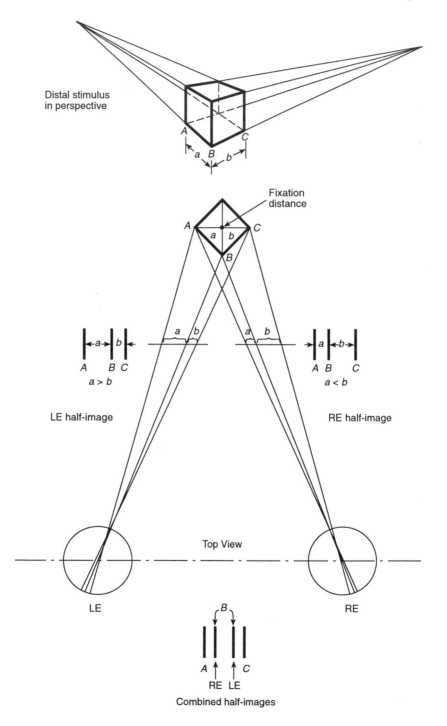

Distal stimulus
in perspective

Fixation
distance

LE half-image

$a > b$

RE half-image

$a < b$

Top View

LE

RE

Combined half-images

view of the eyes and the cube. The proximal patterns produced by the vertical edges are illustrated in the two *half-images* (the horizontal edges are described in figure 4.2). The left-eye half-image is the image seen with the left eye alone and the right-eye half-image is the image seen by the right eye alone.

The vertical outer edges of the cube (sides *A* and *C*) are in a fronto-parallel plane. The fixation point is in this plane, midway between *A* and *C* and behind edge *B*. Thus, edges *A* and *C* are on the horopter and stimulate corresponding retinal points in the two eyes. Edge *B* is closer to the viewer than the horopter. Therefore it produces a crossed disparity represented by the relative positions of edge *B* in the two half-images. The distance between edges *A* and *B* is greater than the distance between edges *B* and *C* (*a* > *b*) in the left eye and is smaller in the right eye (*a* < *b*). Thus, in the left-eye half-image, the representation of contour *B* is shifted to the right and, in the right-eye half-image, it is shifted to the left, a crossed disparity.

If edges *A* and *C* in the two half-images are superimposed, respectively, they may be represented in a single diagram of the combined half-images. Such a diagram is illustrated in the lower portion of the figure. In this diagram, edges *A* and *C* fall on corresponding points and are represented only once. Edge *B* falls on noncorresponding points and, therefore, is represented twice (the representations are identified by the eye they stimulate). Because the right-eye representation of *B* is on the left, and the left-eye representation is on the right, the diagram represents a crossed disparity. When the two half-images are viewed in a stereoscope, edge *B* appears to be closer than *A* and *C*, and the cube appears to be solid.

Differential Perspective

Figure 4.2 illustrates the differences in the two half-images for the horizontal edges. The representation is exaggerated to make the differences easily

Figure 4.1
Contour or edge disparity produced by the vertical edges of a cube directly in front of a viewer. Edges *A* and *C* are on the horopter. Edge *B*, closer to the viewer than the horopter, produces a crossed disparity in the proximal pattern. The two half-images illustrate the difference in the proximal patterns in the two eyes: In the left eye, the distance between edges *A* and *B* is greater than the distance between edges *B* and *C* (*a* > *b*). In the right eye the distance between edges *A* and *B* is less than the distance between edges *B* and *C* (*a* < *b*).

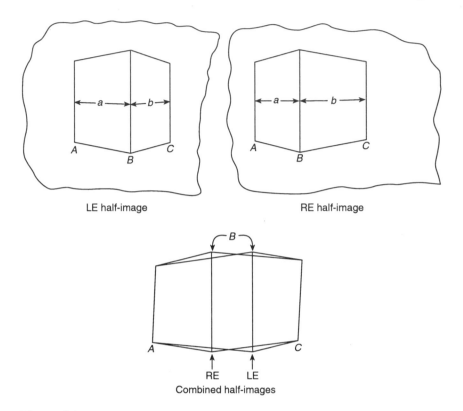

LE half-image   RE half-image

Combined half-images

Figure 4.2
Effects of differential perspective in the two half-images. The horizontal sides
produce vertical disparities (observable in the combined half-images). Vertical edge
B, slightly closer to the viewer than edges *A* and *C*, produces a slightly larger
proximal size.

visible. The figure shows the left- and right-eye half-images for the complete cube as well as the combined half-image. The perspective projections
of the outline shapes of the faces of the cube are different for the two eyes
because the eyes are in different positions in space (see chapter 7). There
are two major consequences of these differences. First, the projective shapes
of the respective sides differ slightly in the two eyes, resulting in a vertical
disparity between the respective horizontal edges. Second, the projection
of edge *B* is slightly larger on the two retinas than those of edges *A* and *C*
because *B* is slightly closer to the viewer. These differences are readily
apparent in the combined half-image.

Binocular Interposition

Interposition (sometimes called *overlay, occlusion* or *superposition*) is most easily understood for monocular vision (see chapter 7 and figure 7.3). *Monocular interposition* describes the fact that a near object occludes a portion of a more distant object in the monocular proximal stimulus. *Binocular interposition* describes the fact that an object is blocked differently in the two eyes by another object in front of it (see figure 3.1). In the proximal representation of an occluded surface, binocular interposition occurs in regions that stimulate one eye and not the other.

Because the eyes view a scene from different positions in space, the occlusion patterns in the two proximal half-images are different (Gulick & Lawson, 1976). This difference is binocular interposition information that can be observed by comparing two stereograms developed by Gulick and Lawson (1976). The first stereogram, illustrated in figure 4.3, does not contain binocular interposition. It is a stereogram containing two squares of dots with a crossed disparity, i.e., the center square is offset to the right in the left-eye half-image and to the left in the right-eye half-image. The relative positions of the inner and outer squares in the stereograms leave blank spaces between the left sides of the dot squares in the left eye and on the right sides of the squares in the right eye (the columns over the arrows).

When viewed stereoscopically, this stimulus results in the perception of two square configurations of dots floating in space at different distances from the viewer (Gulick & Lawson, 1976). Because the smaller square carries a crossed disparity, it appears closer to the viewer than the larger square. However, the dots do not appear to be embedded in a surface. Instead, the elements of the squares appear to be separate dots floating in space, arranged in square patterns. Gulick and Lawson concluded, therefore, that retinal disparity is necessary for the perception of a relative depth difference but is not sufficient for the perception of surface or contour.

Figure 4.4 shows a stereogram that contains binocular interposition information. It is the same as the stereogram in figure 4.3 except that the columns above the arrows are now filled with dots. This stereogram produces the perception of a blank surface with contours in front of a surface filled with dots (Gulick & Lawson, 1976). The nearer surface appears to occlude (cut off from view) the more distant surface. The left eye views the rear surface of dots around the left side of the near surface. Therefore, it is

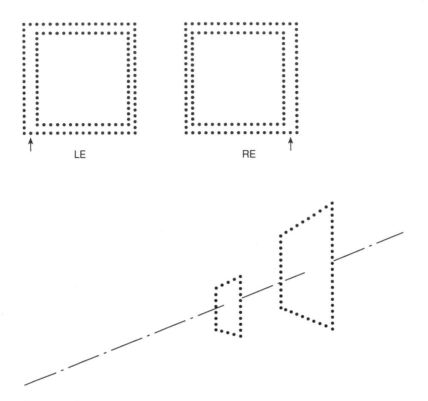

Figure 4.3
A stereogram that contains only retinal disparity. There is no binocular interposition information because the columns above the arrows are empty. When viewed in a stereoscope, the two squares of dots appear to be in different depth planes but there are no contours or surfaces. (From HUMAN STEREOPSIS by W. Lawrence Gulick and Robert B. Lawson. Copyright © 1976 by Oxford University Press, Inc. Used by permission of Oxford University Press, Inc.)

stimulated by three columns of dots on the left side and two columns on the right side. The right eye views the rear surface of dots around the right side of the near surface. Therefore, it is stimulated by three columns of dots on the right side and two columns on the left side. The filled columns of dots over the arrows supply this binocular interposition information about the differential occlusion patterns of the two eyes. Thus, Gulick and Lawson concluded that stereo half-images must contain binocular interposition information as well as retinal disparity in order to produce the perception of surfaces with contours at different relative distances.

   This series of experiments demonstrates clearly that the perception of stereoscopic depth, contour, and surface are emergent qualities in percep-

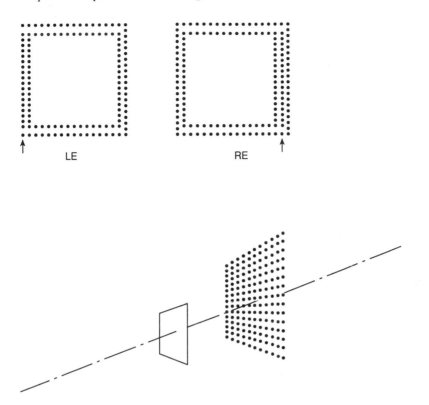

Figure 4.4
Because the space over the arrows is filled with a column of dots, this stereogram contains retinal disparity and binocular interposition. It produces the perception of a homogeneous surface with contours in front of a surface filled with dots. (From HUMAN STEREOPSIS by W. Lawrence Gulick and Robert B. Lawson. Copyright © 1976 by Oxford University Press, Inc. Used by permission of Oxford University Press, Inc.)

tion. That is, they are properties of perception that are not (necessarily) properties of the proximal stimulus. These relationships help in understanding the operation of the perceptual system in general: The proximal input initiates the activity of the perceptual system. The activity of the system produces the emergent qualities in our experience of visual space.

Gradient of Binocular Disparity
Gibson's (1950a, 1966) approach to binocular vision is different from the analysis presented thus far. However, to understand Gibson's theory, it is necessary to comprehend his analysis of gradients in the ambient optic array.

These concepts are described in detail in the section on static monocular perception (chapter 7). A brief description of Gibson's conception of binocular disparity gradients is included here as a contrast to the conventional view.

Gibson noted that distal objects are arrayed continuously in depth over a textured ground surface. Therefore, except for the portion of the visual field stimulated by points on the horopter, the entire binocular field is stimulated by double images. Gibson described this stimulus as a *gradient of retinal disparity,* a gradient that shifts as the eyes move from one fixation to another. For a given fixation, the relative position in depth between the horopter and a point in the optic array determines the direction (crossed or uncrossed) and amount of disparity for that point. In the binocular optic array, the amount of disparity varies directly with distance from the horopter.

For a given fixation, the disparity gradient provides a scale of perceived space in terms of direction and amount of disparity. Direction refers to the relative position in perceived depth (closer or farther away) with respect to the fixation distance, a quality that is determined by the sign of the disparity. The amount of retinal disparity determines the perceived distance from fixation distance. Thus, the part of the field stimulated by an increasing disparity gradient results in the impression of a surface increasing in depth, and the portion of the field stimulated by a decreasing disparity gradient results in the impression of a surface decreasing in depth. Recall, moreover, that the inclination of the horopter means that all objects in the ground plane have zero disparity, since the horopter passes roughly through the feet. Thus, the depth gradient of the ground is obtained from zero disparities (Tyler, 1991b).

Perceptual Outcomes from Traditional Stereograms

Ogle (1950/1964) described the changes in the character of stereoscopic depth perception that correspond to changes in the magnitude of binocular disparity. He also noted that the range of disparity values producing any given type of stereoscopic depth experience increases with increasing peripheral angle.

With small uncrossed disparities, objects appeared single (fusion) and, as disparity increased, they appeared to move progressively behind the fixation point. Ogle described this perceptual experience as fused *patent stereopsis*. As the disparity increased further, fusion was lost, i.e., double images were reported, and the separation between double images increased with increasing disparity. Nevertheless, observers reported experiencing a strong sense of depth despite the fact that the object appeared double. Ogle described this perceptual experience as *obligatory* or *patent stereopsis with double images*. With continued increases of disparity, the observers reported that the vivid impression of depth disappeared, yet the double images appeared unmistakably behind the fixation point. Ogle described this perceptual experience as *qualitative stereopsis*. For disparities larger than those yielding qualitative stereopsis, the double images appeared to be at some unspecifiable distance. Similar regions were found with crossed disparities.

Thus, for patent or qualitative stereopsis, the disparate images can appear fused or not fused, with a depth experience that is vivid and compelling in either case. Within the range of patent stereopsis, the magnitude of the depth response correlates with the magnitude of disparity. However, for larger disparities the depth experience was less obvious and deteriorated with steady fixation. The depth of the double images was apprehended qualitatively, i.e., an observer reported only that the double images appeared "nearer" or "farther" than the fixation point.

Tyler (1983) developed the schematic diagram in figure 4.5 to show how different aspects of the perceptual response vary as a function of binocular disparity. The diagram holds for both crossed and uncrossed disparities. The stereoscopic acuity threshold is the disparity value (near zero) associated with the minimum amount of depth difference that can be discriminated. A stimulus below this threshold is indiscriminable from a flat surface. As disparity increases, there is a region in which perceived depth (perceived distance along the line of sight) is veridical, i.e., it matches the actual depth implied by a given disparity. In the figure, these points fall on the dashed line.

After a certain point, perceived depth falls away from being veridical, suggesting that disparity is not fully processed. There is, nevertheless, an impression of relatively great depth, which increases to a maximum and then decreases as disparity is further increased. At the upper limit, disparity is so great that perceived depth falls to zero. This point may be up to 10 deg of disparity (Richards & Kaye, 1974). The figure also shows Panum's limits of binocular fusion. Disparities smaller than this limit result in the perception of a single fused object in depth; disparities larger than this limit produce diploplia, the image in each eye seen separately, but also in depth.

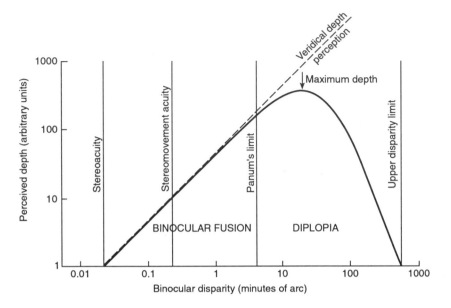

Figure 4.5
The limits of perceived stereoscopic depth and fusion as a function of binocular disparity (Tyler, 1983). The axes are in log units.

In this case, however, depth is not veridical. Nevertheless, the maximum perceivable depth occurs under diplopic conditions.

   Stereoscopic acuity is best in the fovea and decreases toward the periphery. Under normal conditions, we can discriminate a depth difference that produces a disparity of about 10 sec (Westheimer, 1979a; see Collewijn, Steinman, Erkelens, & Regan, 1991, for a review). The best observers reported in the literature achieve 75 percent discrimination close to 2 sec of arc (Tyler, 1983, 1991b). Tyler (1983) translated these values into depth units to illustrate the remarkable accuracy of this system. For close fixation at 10 inches (25.4 cm), the best stereoscopic discrimination produces the perception of a depth difference of one thousandth of an inch (0.001 inches), about one-quarter to one-third the thickness of a human hair (0.003 to 0.004 inches)! For distant fixation at the horizon, we can see that objects two miles away are nearer than the horizon. Thus we can see stereo differences in low cloud formations. This ability represents a *hyperacuity* because the discriminable retinal distances are smaller than the 30 to 35 sec subtense of the smallest foveal cones (Morgan, 1991; Westheimer, 1979b; Wilson, 1991).

Stereoscopic Depth Constancy

The veridical perception of depth produced by retinal disparity is called *stereoscopic depth constancy*. For constancy to occur, retinal disparity must be rescaled when absolute fixation distance changes. To demonstrate stereoscopic constancy, Wallach and Zuckerman (1963) noted that binocular disparity varies according to the square of the distance. A pyramid–shaped object oriented with its apex toward the observer was viewed through a device similar to a mirror stereoscope. In the experimental situation, accommodation and convergence were altered to half the real distance of the pyramid. Wallach and Zuckerman predicted that, when converged at half the original distance, the perceived size of the base would be half the original size but the perceived apex-to-base depth would be one-quarter that of the original. This is essentially what they found. Stereoscopic depth constancy has been demonstrated for viewing distances less than 2 meters (see Ono & Comerford, 1977, for a review). Cormack (1984) reported evidence that apparent depth from stereopsis was veridical beyond 100 meters and that stereo depth could be perceived up to 7.8 km without diploplia.

Dichoptic Stimulation

When different stimuli fall on corresponding points in the two eyes, the stimulus is described as *dichoptic*. The perception that results from dichoptic stimulation depends on the degree of difference between the stimuli in the two eyes. If the difference is small, the result may be perceived depth with fusion or with diploplia. If the difference is large, the most common percepts are binocular mixture, binocular rivalry and suppression, and binocular luster, although double images may be seen without depth.

Binocular Rivalry, Suppression, and Luster

Different stimuli in corresponding areas of the two eyes may be mixed in the perceptual outcome. This result usually occurs when a uniform field in part of one eye contains a detailed stimulus in the corresponding part of the other eye. Stimulation of corresponding proximal regions of the two eyes by very different high-contrast images results in *binocular rivalry*. Rivalry is the antithesis of fusion. Instead of fusion, the two monocular images may alternate repetitively, in whole or in part, with the unseen portion somehow *suppressed* (Levelt, 1968). The alternation may continue as long as the stimuli

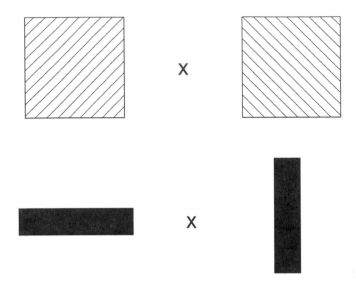

X

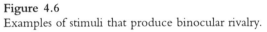

X

Figure 4.6
Examples of stimuli that produce binocular rivalry.

are present and the temporal sequence may be irregular. *Binocular luster* represents a different resolution. It occurs in areas of uniform illumination in which the luminance or color is different in the two eyes. In this response, the images are stable and fused, but appear to be shimmering or lustrous and cannot be localized in depth (Tyler, 1983).

Some stimuli that produce binocular rivalry are illustrated in figure 4.6. For small stimuli (about 1 deg or less), rivalry is usually complete in the sense that the image in one eye is either entirely perceived or not seen at all. In contrast, large stimuli tend to be suppressed in piecemeal fashion (Blake, Fox, & Westendorf, 1974; Blake, O'Shea, & Mueller, 1991). Rivalry can also be produced by differences in contour orientation, contour length, and stimulus size, brightness, or hue. The existence of binocular rivalry demonstrates that, in addition to (or as a consequence of) its fusional activity, the binocular system has an inhibitory component strong enough to act on stimuli that are well above threshold (Fox, 1991).

Summary

This chapter described the stimulus components of traditional stereograms: binocular disparity of (vertical) contours, differential perspective, and differential occlusion (binocular interposition). Traditional stereograms produce the perception of solid objects arrayed in 3D space. They demonstrate stereoscopic depth constancy where perceived depth changes appropriately with changes in retinal disparity. When the half-images are very different, binocular rivalry or suppression may result. The perception may alternate between left- and right-eye views or the object may appear lustrous or shimmering.

5

Cyclopean Perception

Until recently, the patterns used in the study of stereoscopic perception produced disparity of contours or edges when viewed in a stereoscope. Ames's *leaf room* demonstration (Ames, 1955; Ittelson, 1952) was an early attempt to separate binocular disparity from the information supplied monocularly by contours and shapes. The interior walls of the leaf room were made from wire mesh covered with oak leaves (except for one open side), which essentially camouflaged its rectangular shape. When the room was viewed through lenses that changed the binocular disparities, the shape of the room changed accordingly. Although Ames' demonstration was powerful, its impact on research was limited. The resurgence of interest in binocular space perception was sparked by the invention of the random-dot stereogram (Julesz, 1960).

Random-Dot Stereograms

Julesz (1960) constructed stereograms from a textured pattern of dots randomly positioned in a matrix of cells. The *random-dot stereogram* (RDS) contained no lines, contours, or edges that could supply monocular information about the shape of the target figure. In an RDS, each eye is presented with a field of randomly distributed dots that essentially disguise the disparity information it provides when the stereogram is viewed dichoptically at the proper fixation distance. Therefore, using RDSs, retinal disparity could be studied independently, i.e., without interference from knowledge of the shape of the global stereo figure.

To construct an RDS, a random-dot pattern is reproduced so that there is a left and a right half-image. A portion of the pattern in the two half-images is altered so as to carry a retinal disparity of dots. Figure 5.1

0	0	0	1	0	1	1	0	1	0	0	1	1	0	1
1	0	0	0	0	1	0	1	0	1	0	1	1	0	0
0	1	0	1	0	1	1	1	0	0	1	0	0	1	1
0	0	1	1	1	0	0	0	0	1	1	1	0	0	0
0	0	1	1	Y	Y	X	X	X	X	Y	1	0	0	1
1	1	1	1	Y	X	Y	Y	X	Y	X	1	0	1	1
0	1	1	0	Y	X	X	X	Y	Y	Y	1	1	0	1
1	1	1	1	X	X	Y	X	Y	X	X	1	0	0	1
1	1	1	1	Y	Y	Y	Y	X	X	Y	0	0	1	1
1	0	1	0	Y	X	Y	X	X	Y	Y	1	1	0	0
1	0	0	0	X	X	X	Y	X	X	X	1	0	0	1
0	1	1	1	1	0	0	1	0	1	1	0	0	0	1
1	1	0	1	1	0	1	1	0	0	0	1	1	1	0
0	1	1	1	1	1	1	0	0	1	1	0	1	1	0
0	0	1	1	1	1	1	1	0	1	0	1	1	0	0	1

0	0	0	1	0	1	1	0	1	0	0	1	1	0	1
1	0	0	0	0	1	0	1	0	1	0	1	1	0	0
0	1	0	1	0	1	1	1	0	0	1	0	0	1	1
0	0	1	1	1	0	0	0	0	1	1	1	0	0	0
0	0	1	1	Y	X	X	X	X	Y	A	1	0	0	1
1	1	1	1	X	Y	Y	X	Y	X	A	1	0	1	1
0	1	1	0	X	X	X	Y	Y	Y	B	1	1	0	1
1	1	1	1	X	Y	X	Y	X	X	A	1	0	0	1
1	1	1	1	Y	Y	Y	X	X	Y	A	0	0	1	1
1	0	0	0	X	Y	X	X	Y	Y	B	1	1	0	0
1	0	0	0	X	X	Y	X	X	X	B	1	0	0	1
0	1	1	1	1	0	0	1	0	1	1	0	0	0	1
1	1	0	1	1	0	1	1	0	0	0	1	1	1	0
0	1	1	1	1	1	1	0	0	1	1	0	1	1	0
0	0	1	1	1	1	1	0	1	0	1	1	0	0	1

Figure 5.1
Construction of a random-dot stereogram (see text for details).

illustrates the procedure for producing a random–dot stereogram from a 15 ×
15 matrix of cells. The numbers **0** and **1** indicate whether the cells are filled
(black) or empty (white). In the figure, a central square area (7 cells × 7 cells)
has been selected to carry a crossed retinal disparity. The **0**s and **1**s have
been changed to **X**s and **Y**s to identify the pattern within this area. The
pattern in the left-eye half-image is reproduced in the corresponding 7 ×
7-cell matrix in the right-eye half-image. However, the pattern is displaced
one column to the left. Thus, the random–dot patterns in the outer four
rows and columns are exactly the same in the two half-images but the central
patterns are offset horizontally by one column. To complete the right-eye
half-image, the empty column (the fifth column from the right) is filled
with a new random pattern indicated by **A**s and **B**s.

When these half-images are viewed in a stereoscope, the left-eye
half-image stimulates the left eye and the right-eye half-image stimulates
the right eye, producing a horizontal crossed disparity in the central portion
of the random-dot pattern. This stereogram results in the perception of a
square central surface in front of another larger surface. The surfaces appears
to be separated by sharp contours that belong to the central (nearer) surface.

Wallpaper Phenomenon, Autostereogram

In RDSs, the stereoscopic information is captured in the two half-images
that must be presented to each eye separately. In autostereograms, the
stereoscopic information is contained within a single stimulus pattern and

is made effectively dichoptic by shifting fixation to a depth plane off the plane of the stimulus.

The basic principles that operate in autostereograms were known for a long time as the *wallpaper phenomenon,* discovered in the last century by Brewster (see Ittelson, 1960; Mitchison & McKee, 1985, 1987a, 1987b; and Tyler, 1991b, for details). When a viewer fixates a point on a wall containing a horizontally repetitive pattern in the wallpaper, the wall appears to be at the appropriate (veridical) distance. If, however, fixation is in front of or behind the wall in such a way as to cause alternate elements of the repeating pattern to fall within corresponding fusional areas in the two eyes, the wall appears to be in a different depth plane, closer or farther away from the viewer.

Figure 5.2 illustrates the wallpaper phenomenon when the viewer fixates a point closer than the wall. At a particular distance, corresponding points are stimulated by pattern A in the right eye and pattern B in the left eye. This stimulus is perceived as a single pattern a-b in the plane of the fixated distance. These relationships hold for the entire repetitive pattern so that the wall is seen at the fixated distance. Similar relationships hold for fixation distances beyond the wall.

The wallpaper phenomenon illustrates the basic disparity relationships used to construct an *autostereogram.* Any repetitive pattern may appear at different depth planes depending on the convergence of the eyes. In the autostereogram, the stereoscopic information is represented by a repetition of a random pattern (Tyler & Chang, 1977). If the eyes converge by the width of one repetition, each random strip will be superimposed dichoptically on an adjacent strip. The stimulus will be perceived in a new depth plane determined by the retinal disparity equal to the separation width on the original stimulus plane. In this way, any perceived surface in depth can be created by varying the repetition width at each point. Autostereograms permit free viewing, i.e., viewing without the use of stereoscopes or other devices, because the stereoscopic information is coded in repeated patterns rather than half-images. They requires only a single random-dot field to camouflage the shape information so there is no limit to their size (see Tyler, 1983, 1991b, for details).

Figure 5.3 contains a random-dot autostereogram of a checkerboard pattern. To view this stereogram, hold it about 16 inches (approximately 40 cm) away and fixate an object about 2 inches (about 5 cm) in front of the page. A 3D perception of the checkerboard will slowly emerge. It might

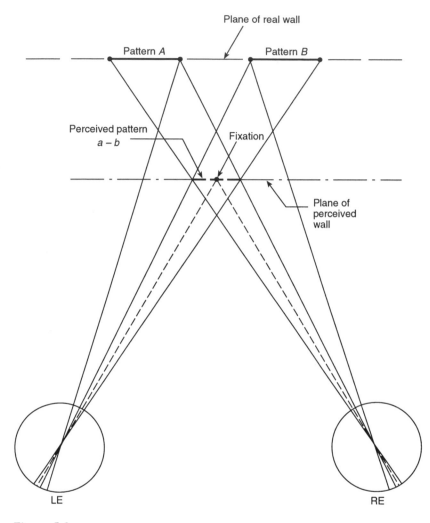

Figure 5.2
The wallpaper phenomenon. The wall contains a wallpaper pattern that repeats horizontally. When a viewer fixates a point closer than the wall and fuses alternate patterns *(A* and *B)*, the perceived pattern (a–b) appears to be in the plane of the fixation point, i.e., at a different location in depth.

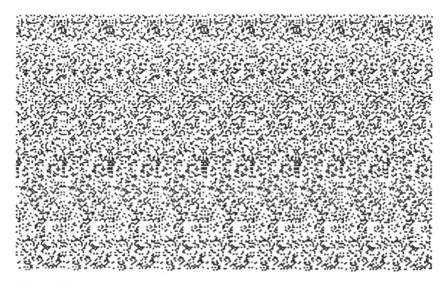

Figure 5.3
A random-dot autostereogram of a checkerboard pattern (Tyler, 1991a). To view this stereogram, hold it about 16 inches (approximately 40 cm) away and fixate your finger about 2 inches (about 5 cm) in front of the page.

take a little time and practice before the 3D pattern is perceived. When the checkerboard appears, the fixated object can be removed, and the entire field can be observed without losing the 3D effect.

Stereoscopic Contours

The advantage of studying stereopsis using random-dot stereograms or autostereograms is that the stimulus displays are devoid of contour, shape, and familiarity information about the stimulus object. The stimulus surface is textured with random dots, making it effectively indistinguishable from the rest of the surface. The disparity information is carried by the patterns in the dots rather than by edges. Julesz suggested, therefore, that contours are not necessary for the perception of stereoscopic depth, i.e., monocular processing of form is not a prerequisite to stereoscopic form perception. This proposal refutes the hypothesis that stereoscopic depth perception depends on the disparity of identical contours in the proximal half-images, the generally accepted view until the 1960s (see Julesz, 1971, 1986, and Tyler, 1991a, 1991b, for reviews).

Furthermore, these stimuli can produce the perception of contours despite the fact that there are no contours in the stimulus. Both RDSs and autostereograms produce the perception of 3D objects whose edges appear as clearly defined contours. For example, using the stereogram in figure 5.4, Gulick and Lawson (1976) showed dramatically that the perception of stereoscopic depth gives rise to the perception of surfaces and contours. The stereogram was constructed from a matrix of large dots with a disparate submatrix defined by the omission of dots. The figure shows a surround matrix with all the dots filled (100 percent matrix density) and a shifted blank central submatrix (no dots filled or 0 percent matrix density). When viewed stereoscopically, the homogeneous (central) area of the submatrix appeared to be a surface, positioned in space between the observer and the plane of the surface containing the dots. The near surface appeared to mask from view a portion of the rear surface. Furthermore, this occluding surface appeared to have sharp contours on all sides located inside the boundary

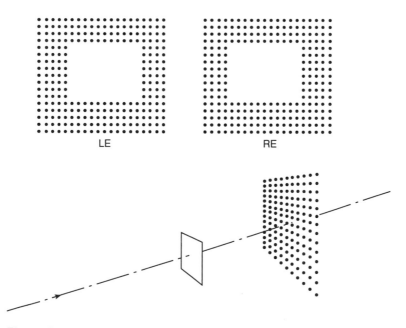

Figure 5.4
A stereogram constructed by selective omission of dots. It produces the perception of a homogeneous occluding surface with contours. (From HUMAN STEREOPSIS by W. Lawrence Gulick and Robert B. Lawson. Copyright © 1976 by Oxford University Press, Inc. Used by permission of Oxford University Press, Inc.)

rows and columns, despite the fact that the stereo half-images contained no monocular contours.

The perceived contours produced by RDSs, autostereograms, and large-dot stereograms are edges or borders of surfaces that arise from stereo-scopic processing. They are not produced by contours in the proximal stimulus. This sequence reverses the relationships between contours and depth perception—instead of disparity of contours in the proximal stimulus giving rise to relative depth in perception, contours in perception are now seen as a result of the perception of relative depth due to stereopsis (Gulick & Lawson, 1976; Julesz, 1960, 1971; Lawson & Gulick, 1967).

Stereo Contours in Homogeneous Space

The stereoscopic contours described thus far appear adjacent to dots in the stimulus and follow the positions of the dots closely. Gulick and Lawson (1976) devised the stereogram in figure 5.5 to produce the perception of an occluding surface whose contours are not adjacent to the dots carrying

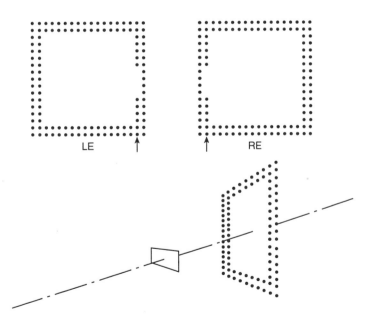

Figure 5.5
A stereogram that produces the perception of an occluding surface whose contours are not adjacent to the dots carrying the disparity. (From HUMAN STEREOPSIS by W. Lawrence Gulick and Robert B. Lawson. Copyright © 1976 by Oxford University Press, Inc. Used by permission of Oxford University Press, Inc.)

the disparity. In this stereogram, the stereoscopic information is carried by the absence of dots in the columns indicated by the arrows. In the left-eye half-image, there is a discontinuity in the right side of the dot pattern of the inner square and, in the right-eye half-image, there is a discontinuity in the left side of the dot pattern of the inner square.

When the stereogram was viewed stereoscopically, a small rectangular surface appeared to be floating in space, closer to the viewer than a larger surface containing two adjacent squares of dots. The lateral ends of the near surface differentially occluded a portion of the inner square. The horizontal edges of this surface appeared in the central area of the visual field that contained no stimulus, an area that Gulick and Lawson called *homogeneous space*. Thus, stereoscopic contours do not always appear adjacent to pattern elements.

The subjective contours described thus far have all been straight lines. Gulick and Lawson (1976) constructed the stereogram illustrated in figure 5.6 to determine whether these contours were always straight lines or might also be curved. The stereoscopic information in the upper portion of the stereogram is carried by a continuous circular contour. In the lower portion, the information is carried by a matrix of dots spaced to permit completion of the figure as a regular octagon, a figure with straight contours. Gulick and Lawson reasoned that, if the perceptual system works according to Gestalt organizing principles (see chapter 7), the circle in the upper portion of the stereogram would be completed by a circular contour in the lower portion. When viewed stereoscopically, the lower portion of the stimulus was seen as an octagon, suggesting that straight-line contours have primacy in stereoscopic vision. Gulick and Lawson found that curved contours appear only when the interposed surfaces must have curved boundaries to account for the differences in the half-images.

Two Mechanisms for Stereoscopic Depth

Since forms or shapes are not present in RDSs and autostereograms, stereoscopic form cannot be represented in the processing sequence until the representation of information from the two eyes comes together (Julesz, 1960, 1971). The *cyclopean level* of processing is where this occurs, and the term *cyclopean* may be applied to any part of the stimulus that is not visible monocularly but is visible stereoscopically, i.e., when disparity processing is involved. (This usage should not be confused with the *cyclopean eye,* from

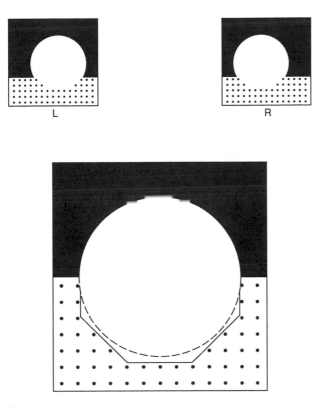

Figure 5.6
A stereogram used to determine whether perceived stereoscopic contours are always straight lines or may also be curved. (From HUMAN STEREOPSIS by W. Lawrence Gulick and Robert B. Lawson. Copyright © 1976 by Oxford University Press, Inc. Used by permission of Oxford University Press, Inc.)

which we experience visual directions). The difference between cyclopean and noncyclopean (traditional) stereograms suggests that form processing in RDSs may be different from that involved in traditional stereograms and in the recognition of form monocularly.

Shimojo and Nakajima (1981) obtained more direct experimental evidence that the processes involved in viewing traditional stereograms with form disparity are different from those involved in viewing cyclopean stereograms. They wore spectacles that reversed binocular disparity and vergence information. The device was worn continuously for nine days during which stereoscopic perception was tested with random-dot stereograms and contour-disparity stereograms. The noncyclopean stereograms resulted in a reversed perceived depth direction with long-lasting after-

effects. The random-dot stereograms did not produce the reversal of perceived stereoscopic depth and there was no adaptive change. This finding
supports the view that the two types of stereograms activated two different
processes. It also implies that the perception of form from random-dot
stereograms might be a different process from that involved in the recognition of monocular forms in contour stereograms (Tyler, 1991b).

Local versus Global Disparity Ranges

When the disparity in one location of the visual field is processed without
reference to the disparities in other locations, or to other disparities in the
same location, the process is described as *local* and defines a local disparity
range. In contrast, processes that require interaction between local disparity
processing mechanisms are described as *global* and define the global processing range. Global processing appears to be limited to small disparities
whereas local processing apparently applies to both large and small disparities
(see Tyler, 1991b, for details).

Fine versus Coarse Disparities

The distinction between fine and coarse disparities in cyclopean vision from
RDSs is independent of the distinction between local and global disparity
ranges. It is similar to Ogle's (1950/1964) separation of patent and qualitative
stereopsis in response to contour disparities (see chapter 4). Recall that
patent stereopsis is produced by small disparities and perceived depth is
linearly proportional to the magnitude of the disparity. Qualitative stereopsis
is produced by large disparities and perceived depth is related only to the
sign of the disparity. The difference is that Panum's areas do not exist for
cyclopean vision from RDSs. The concept of Panum's limit describes a
property of the mechanism that resolves horizontal and vertical contour
disparities to produce fusion or diplopia. In contrast, RDSs do not produce
diplopia no matter how large the disparity.

Pyknostereopsis and Diastereopsis

A similar distinction can be made between two types of responses in the
cyclopean domain. An RDS can be constructed that contains two overlaid
disparity planes with a disparity separation between them. When the disparity separation is small, the two planes in the stimulus are fused in
perception—they appear to be a single dense plane. This perception is
pyknostereopsis (from the Greek for "dense"). Within the pykno range, there

is averaging of the depth of the component stimulus planes. With a large disparity separation between the stimulus planes, two separate transparent surfaces are seen in two different depth planes. This perception is *diastereopsis* (from the Greek for "separate" or "transparent"). The two transparent planes are equivalent to the 3D images in diploplia because they are coexistent diaphanous surfaces.

Cyclopean Disparity Limits

Figure 5.7 shows Tyler's (1991b) schematic overview of cyclopean disparity limits with perceived depth plotted as a function of binocular disparity. The lower end of the function is similar to that for noncyclopean disparity illustrated in figure 4.5, although the threshold of cyclopean stereoacuity is higher, typically about 20 to 40 sec (Akerstrom & Todd, 1988; Schumer, 1979). Below this limit, binocular disparity produces perceptions that cannot be differentiated from a flat surface; above this limit, perceived depth increases veridically with increases in disparity. The line representing the depth fusion limit is the disparity value where pyknostereopsis changes to diastereopsis. This line is at approximately 20 to 30 min of arc. Diastereopsis drops to zero at the upper limit, up to 2 deg of cyclopean disparity depending on the stimulus (Tyler, 1991b; Tyler & Julesz, 1976).

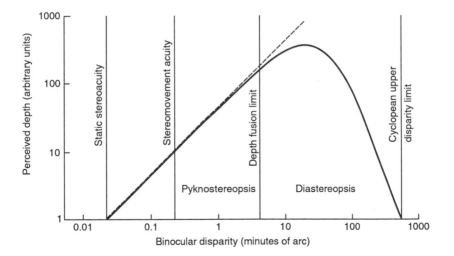

Figure 5.7
Schematic diagram showing cyclopean limits of perceived depth and fusion (Tyler, 1991b). The axes are in log units.

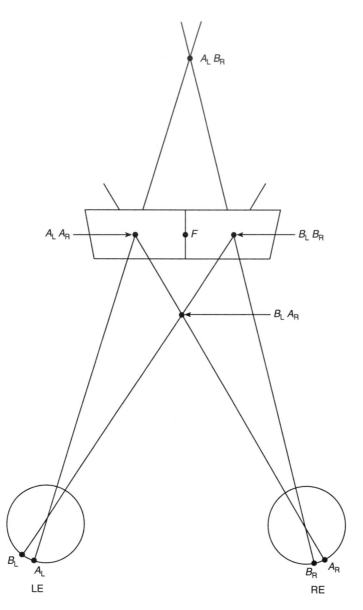

Figure 5.8

The correspondence problem in binocular vision illustrated for two distal points, A and B. The "true" correspondence is A_L-A_R and B_L-B_R. But there are also false target locations that produce "false" correspondences B_L-A_R and A_L-B_R.

Computational Theories, Correspondence Problem

The development of RDSs brought renewed interest in the *correspondence problem,* the problem of determining corresponding points in the two eyes. The solution to the correspondence problem describes how to determine the point in one eye that is the "true" match for a particular point in the other eye (in the sense that it leads to veridical perception). Determining correspondence is a difficult problem because there are many spurious matches between similar features in the respective eyes. The problem is illustrated in figure 5.8 for two adjacent distal points, A and B. The "true" correspondence is A_L-A_R and B_L-B_R. But there are also false target locations that produce "false" correspondences B_L-A_R and A_L-B_R. Computational theorists have proposed algorithms for solving the correspondence problem to extract depth from disparate images. The variety and complexity of these theories put this topic beyond the scope of this book (see Foley, 1991; Tyler, 1991b; and Weinshall & Malik, 1994, for details).

Summary

This chapter described the random-dot stereogram and the autostereogram, two ways of presenting camouflaged stereoscopic information. Both stimuli produce the perception of surfaces with contours in different depth planes. The characteristics of perceptions produced by these stimuli suggest that there are different processes activated by traditional and random-dot stimuli.

II

Monocular Perception

The discussion of monocular space perception begins in chapter 6 with the issue of stimulus inadequacy, which raises the fundamental question about the amount of information in the proximal stimulus. Chapter 7 describes the information in pictorial cues and oculomotor adjustments, as well as the outcomes of automatic organizing processes. The empiricist view is discussed in chapter 8 in the context of analyzing perceived size and distance and the related invariance hypotheses. Chapter 9 introduces Gibson's psychophysical view and the concept of optical texture gradient.

The remaining chapters focus on the analysis of motion of objects and of observers. Chapter 10 describes lateral or parallactic motion and introduces the optical flow field. Chapter 11 describes the perception of motion in depth (radial motion) of rigid objects. Chapter 12 describes the perception of objects rotating in space and the kinetic depth effect. Johansson's vector analysis is described in this context. Finally, chapter 13 describes models of motion detectors and some supporting evidence.

6

Stimulus Inadequacy: The Fundamental Problem of Monocular Perception

As in binocular space perception, the distal-proximal relationships involved in monocular space perception are described by geometrical optics. Nevertheless, the analysis of proximal-perceptual relations has been formulated in two ways, differing in whether the stimulus contains enough information to determine a particular perceptual response uniquely.

The classical empiricist position (Ames, 1955; Berkeley, 1709/1963; Brunswick, 1956; Helmholtz, 1866/1963; Rock, 1977) rests on the argument that the proximal stimulus does not contain enough information to determine a unique perception. This is the argument for stimulus inadequacy (see Runeson, 1988, for a detailed critique of the notion of stimulus inadequacy). The alternative position argues that the stimulus appears to be inadequate only when it is analyzed into small units (Gibson, 1950a, 1966). These two views of the stimulus have produced three major types of theories: the empiricist view, the psychophysical view, and a third view that attributes a major role to automatic activity of the perceptual system itself.

Stimulus Inadequacy

Stimulus inadequacy applies to all aspects of input information. In this section, the concept is illustrated using perceived size.

Visual Angle

Figure 6.1 shows a distal edge in the frontal plane of a viewer at point P. The line is represented by a vertical arrow of size S, its physical size, at a distance D from the viewer. Light reflected from the edge impinges on the retina. This retinal extent is the proximal stimulus. The size of the proximal stimulus is conveniently specified in terms of the *visual angle* α, the angle

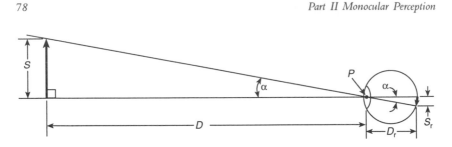

Figure 6.1
A distal edge of size S at a distance D from the viewer at point P. The size of the stimulus is specified in terms of the *visual angle* α, where tan $\alpha = S/D$.

made at the eye by the envelope of light reflected from the arrow. By geometrical optics: tan $\alpha = S_r/D_r$; where S_r is *retinal size*, D_r is the distance between the nodal point and the retina (a constant), and α is the visual angle. Thus, S_r varies directly with tan α, and tan α is a function of S and D:

$$\tan \alpha = S/D. \tag{6.1}$$

With D, constant, visual angle represents the linear extent of stimulation on the receptor surface. For most objects, visual angle is small (less than 10 deg) and tan α approximates α, yielding:

$$\alpha = S/D. \tag{6.2}$$

These quantities represent physical measurements where S is a property of the distal object and D is a property of the space between the distal object and the viewer. Therefore, S and D are independent, and visual angle varies directly with S and inversely with D. Thus, the proximal stimulus produced by a distal edge can be specified by the visual angle.

Figure 6.2 illustrates the distal-proximal relationships for a line slanted toward the viewer. The slant angle (δ) is measured from the vertical, and A represents the vertical distance of the near end. If D represents the distance from the viewer to the far end of the line, there is a small difference (ΔD) in the distance between the near and far ends. From equation 6.1: tan $\alpha = A/(D - \Delta D)$. Substitute $\Delta D = S \sin \delta$ and $A = S \cos \delta$ to get the visual angle subtense:

$$\tan \alpha = S(\cos \delta)/[D - S(\sin \delta)]. \tag{6.3}$$

Equivalent Configurations
Figure 6.3 shows a single contour of size S at a distance D from a viewer at P. This contour subtends a visual angle α at the eye of the viewer. It is

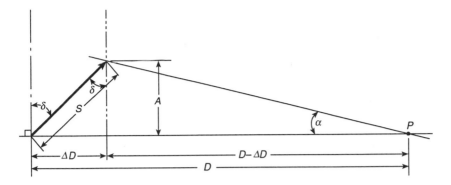

Figure 6.2
A line slanted toward the viewer. The slant angle (δ) is measured from the vertical. If D is the distance from the viewer to the far end of the line and ΔD is the difference in distance between the ends, $\tan \alpha = S(\cos \delta)/[D - S(\sin \delta)]$.

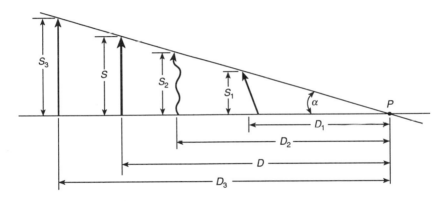

Figure 6.3
A contour of size S at a distance D from a viewer at P subtends a visual angle α at the eye of the viewer. Many other distal edges could produce the same proximal stimulus, for example, objects of sizes S_1, S_2, or S_3 at appropriate distances D_1, D_2, and D_3.

clear that there are many other distal edges that could produce the same proximal stimulus. Indeed, for any given stimulus at the eye (visual angle = α), there are many objects that produce the same visual angle. For example, objects of sizes S_1, S_2, S_3, etc., subtend the same visual angle provided they are placed at the appropriate distances (D_1, D_2, D_3, etc.). Furthermore, these lines may represent edges or contours that are straight or wavy, vertical or slanted. The only restriction is that they remain within the envelope of light described by the visual angle.

One could argue, moreover, that there is an infinite number of distal lines that could produce the same visual angle as the lines in figure 6.3. In this sense there is a collection of distal objects that could produce the same proximal stimulus, a family of *equivalent configurations* (Ittelson, 1960). Two or more members of the same family of equivalent configurations produce the same proximal stimulus and, therefore, supply the same information at the eye. The fact that it is possible to describe families of equivalent configurations suggests that the stimulus array does not contain enough information to determine a unique percept. That is, the proximal stimulus is inadequate.

A similar analysis can be made for surfaces at different slants. Figure 6.4 illustrates this by showing a number of different surfaces at different slants, all of which subtend the same solid visual angle, α by β, at P, the position of the viewer.

Invariance, Noninvariance, and Constancy

If the stimulus is inadequate, the problem of space perception becomes one of discovering how additional processing produces unique perceptual experiences. For a given proximal pattern, the possible perceptions may be divided into two broad classes: invariance and noninvariance outcomes. *Invariance* describes perceptions that correspond to the physical objects that could have produced the proximal stimulus, i.e., to members of the family of equivalent configurations associated with that particular proximal stimulus. *Noninvariance* describes perceptions that are not members of the family of equivalent configurations producing the particular proximal stimulus.

Perceptual constancy is one common invariance outcome that has been intensively investigated (see Epstein, 1977a, for history and detailed discussion of constancy). Perceptual constancy occurs when, despite changes in

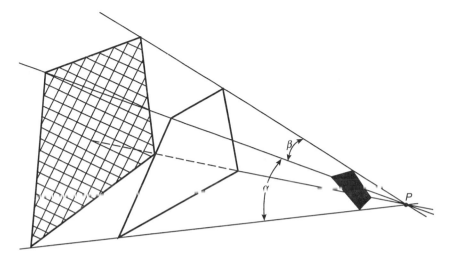

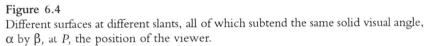

Figure 6.4
Different surfaces at different slants, all of which subtend the same solid visual angle, α by β, at *P*, the position of the viewer.

the proximal stimulus, the perceived object corresponds to the specific distal object that is producing the proximal stimulus. For example, when a rigid object is placed in different positions or orientations in depth, the proximal pattern it produces changes in size and/or shape. Nevertheless, the object appears to remain the same in size and shape, a perceptual experience described as size or shape constancy.

If an object moves continuously, the proximal pattern changes continuously. Once again, perceptual constancy means that, despite these changes in the proximal stimulus, the object appears to be constant in size and shape, a property sometimes described as *perceived rigidity*. The same relations hold when the viewer moves. Constancy is a common perceptual experience, an outcome described by saying that perception is *veridical* or true to life. Indeed, constancy may be the essential problem in the study of visual space perception.

Three Kinds of Theories

The way stimulus inadequacy is treated leads directly to different types of theories. The three major views are introduced here to set the stage for more detailed discussions in subsequent chapters.

Empiricist (Helmholtzian) View

The empiricist view starts with stimulus inadequacy and suggests that the input must be supplemented by learning, memory, inference, assumptions, computations, or other processes that frequently resemble cognitive or inferential processes (Rock, 1977, 1983; Wallach, 1976, 1984). In this view, for example, information about distance may be "taken into account" by the application of rules or algorithms whose outcomes appear to be logical or rational (Epstein, 1973; Rock, 1977).

The empiricist position can be further differentiated according to the role assigned to the proximal stimulus. Some empiricists (e.g., Rock, 1977; Rock & Kaufman, 1962) assert that the proximal stimulus sets the limits for possible perceptions. That is, the perception must be a member of the family of equivalent configurations determined by the proximal stimulus. Another group (primarily the students and colleagues of Ames, sometimes called *transactionalists*), believes that perception is not limited by the proximal stimulus (Ames, 1955; Ittelson, 1952, 1960, 1968). For this group, perception is determined by the global stimulus pattern and the past experience of the viewer, and is not constrained by a particular local aspect of the proximal input.

Psychophysical (Gibsonian) View

Gibson (1950a, 1966) proposed that the natural stimulus contains a great deal of information. Stimulation only appears to be inadequate because it is brought into the laboratory and analyzed in such detail that the appropriate stimulus variables can no longer be identified. To Gibson, the natural stimulus contains all the information necessary to determine 3D perception directly. In this view, it should be possible to discover higher-order stimulus variables that correlate with various aspects of 3D perception and, therefore, perception can be described as a direct representation of these complex stimuli. That is why Gibson's view is sometimes called a *theory of direct perception*.

Automatic Perceptual System Activity

The proponents of this view believe that perception results from proximal stimulus input (simple or complex) and *automatic processing activity* of the perceptual system. For the Gestalt psychologists, automatic perceptual system activity was described by organizational principles or laws (Koffka, 1935; see Beck, 1982, for various modern interpretations of the Gestalt

view). Johansson (1950, 1977; Jansson, Burgström, & Epstein, 1994) proposed automatic processes that treat kinetic input as a single rigid unit
moving in 3D space. These processes are activities of the perceptual system
that are automatically activated by specific proximal patterns.

Chair Demonstration

The chair demonstration developed by Ames (1955; Ittelson, 1952, 1960)
illustrates the perceptual problems raised by the relationships described
above. The demonstration consists of the three separate viewing fields
illustrated in figure 6.5. The upper portion of the figure shows the essentials
of one of the fields. The lower portion of the figure shows side views of
the distal configurations in the three viewing fields.

In each field, the support wires are stretched between a small viewing
aperture, *P,* and a back wall painted flat black. One field contains a real
chair made of white strings suspended by thin black wires. The manner in
which this field is constructed is illustrated in the upper portion of the figure.
The vertical back leg, *AB,* is attached to wires *A'P* and *B'P* that are stretched
between the back wall and the viewing aperture at *P.* When an eye is at *P,*
the wires corresponds to the visual angle subtended by leg *AB.* There is a
pair of wires at *P* that corresponds to the visual angle for each leg, respectively, and a simulated seat painted on the back wall that subtends the same
solid visual angle as the space for the seat on the suspended string chair.
When this field is viewed from point *P* or from another position (e.g., from
the side), one sees a white string chair suspended in space.

The other two fields contain sets of black wires in exactly the same
positions stretched between their respective viewing points and the back
wall. In the second field (b), these wires are cut by an imaginary plane
positioned at a slant to the back wall. The legs, seat, and back of the chair
are projected onto this plane, and white strings are tied between pairs of
black wires that correspond to the respective components. Therefore, the
distal stimulus in this field is a 2D projection of the 3D string chair.

In the third field (c), the procedure of the second field is repeated
separately for each component of the chair. For example, the wires for the
back left leg are cut by a plane slanted at a randomly selected angle to the
back wall. A white string is tied to the wires in this plane. Now the wires
for the back right leg are cut with an imaginary plane slanted at a different randomly selected angle to the back wall, and a white string is tied

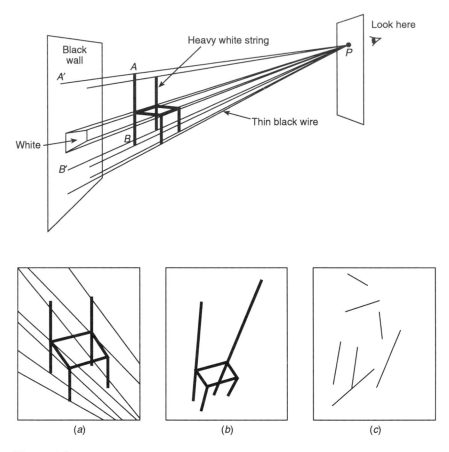

Figure 6.5
The chair demonstration (Ames, 1955; Ittelson, 1952) has three viewing fields. In each field, the support wires are stretched between a small viewing aperture, *P,* and a back wall painted flat black. The lower portion of the figure shows side views of the distal configurations in the three viewing fields (see text for details).

connecting these wires in that plane. This procedure is repeated for all pairs of wires for all components of the chair. Consequently, the distal stimulus for this field is an array of strings suspended in space in an apparently random manner. When viewed from the respective viewing points, however, the proximal stimulus patterns in the three fields are the same. In all three cases, viewers report seeing the same 3D string chair.

The chair demonstration answers a number of questions but also raises some important ones. It illustrates equivalent configurations by demonstrating three different distal collections of lines (strings) that produce the same proximal pattern when viewed from a particular vantage point. It demon-strates the general point that perceptual outcomes are determined by proxi-mal patterns, not distal patterns. That is, we see the same object in all three cases because the proximal stimuli are the same. But this demonstration does not explain why we see a 3D object when the proximal stimulus is flat or why we see a chair rather than some other object. There are many different answers to these questions, most of which are encompassed by the three kinds of theories.

Summary

This chapter began the study of monocular space perception by describing stimulus inadequacy, the proposition that the proximal stimulus does not contain enough information to determine perception uniquely. Three types of theories were described: the empiricist view that the stimulus must be supplemented with other information, frequently from memory or learning; the psychophysical view that higher-order stimulus variables determine perception directly, and the view that the stimulus is organized automatically by processes that are part of the structure of the perceptual system. Each of these views is elaborated in subsequent chapters.

7

Pictorial Cues, Oculomotor Adjustments, Automatic Organizing Processes, and Observer Tendencies

Monocular information in the proximal stimulus can be represented in a frontal plane projection that can be analyzed into separate "cues." This information, described collectively as the *pictorial cues,* is a subset of monocular cues. Artists use the pictorial cues to represent ordinal information about depth in drawings and paintings. Although pictures frequently appear realistic, when viewed individually, pictorial cues are ambiguous in the sense of stimulus inadequacy—they do not determine a unique perceptual outcome.

Pictorial Cues

This section describes the pictorial cues except for visual angle (retinal size). Visual angle has been described in chapter 6 and its theoretical role is analyzed in the next chapter.

Linear Perspective, Outline Shape

Geometrical optics describes the geometry relating distal objects in 3D space to the proximal pattern. However, the proximal pattern itself is described by a different geometry, the geometry of *linear perspective.* Figure 7.1 illustrates this geometry for two perspective representations of an upright rectangular solid. The vertical edges and surfaces are aligned with gravity, and the horizontal edges and surfaces are parallel to the ground, i.e., perpendicular to the direction of gravity.

In figure 7.1a, the center of the object is approximately on a line of sight to the horizon. In the projection, the horizontal edges converge to vanishing points on the horizon on both sides of the object. The projections of the vertical edges are essentially parallel. Figure 7.1b shows the proximal projections of two objects, one above and one below the line of sight to

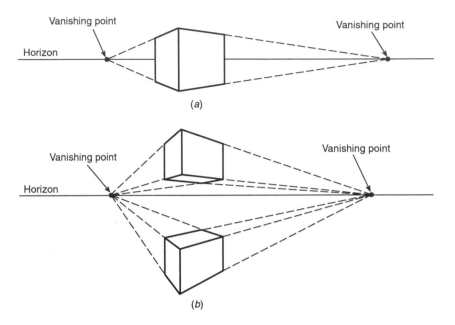

Figure 7.1
Perspective representations of an upright rectangular solid. (a) The center of the
object is approximately on a line of sight to the horizon. (b) Projections of objects
above and below the line of sight.

the horizon. Again the vertical edges are parallel and the horizontal edges
converge toward vanishing points on the horizon. However, in these positions, the top or bottom surfaces of the objects are exposed to view,
depending on the position of the object relative to the horizon and the line
of sight. The horizontal edges of these surfaces converge toward the same
vanishing points as those of the lateral surfaces.

Figure 7.2 shows projections of a single surface in more detail. In figure 7.2a, the outline shape of a square surface is slanted with respect to a
horizontal axis in the frontal plane. In figure 7.2b, a square surface is slanted
with respect to a vertical axis in the frontal plane. In both cases, rotation
around the axis transforms the shape from a square to a trapezoid. The sides
of the square that are perpendicular to the axis of rotation (the sides of the
trapezoid) project as converging lines that meet at a vanishing point.

The sides that are parallel to the axis of rotation remain parallel to it
and to the frontal plane. The edge that was rotated toward the viewer
becomes the base of the trapezoid. This side of the trapezoid is slightly larger
than the corresponding side of the square. The edge that was rotated away

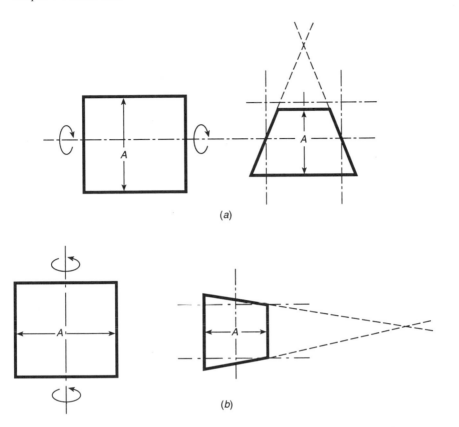

Figure 7.2
Proximal projections of the outline shape of a square surface that is slanted with respect to (a) the horizontal axis or (b) the vertical axis.

from the viewer becomes the upper edge of the trapezoid and is slightly smaller than the corresponding side of the square (see discussion of visual angle in chapter 8). Thus, in the proximal projection, the more distant edge is *foreshortened* with respect to the near edge. The distance between these edges, the *altitude* of the trapezoid A, is also smaller than the corresponding measurement of the square, i.e., the altitude is *compressed*. (The terms *foreshortening* and *compression* are sometimes used interchangeably.) Thus, a distal square at a slant projects as a trapezoid whose altitude is compressed in the direction of the slant.

Relative Size
Relative size refers to the mutual influence of one proximal extent on another proximal extent (Gogel, 1977; Hochberg & Hochberg, 1952; Rock &

Ebenholtz, 1959). Figure 7.2 illustrates one aspect of relative size that is directly tied to linear perspective. When two contours are part of a single outline shape, their relative size can act as a cue to their relative distance. In the figure, the larger side of the trapezoid appears closer than the shorter side.

Relative size can also act as a cue to distance when contours are not connected. For example, Rock and Ebenholtz (1959) presented luminous vertical lines surrounded by luminous rectangles in a dark field. The lines within the surrounds were judged equal in size when they were approximately equal to the same proportions of the heights of their respective frameworks. Rock and Ebenholtz concluded that the perceived size of a line was determined by the relationship between the angular extent of the line to that of the surround.

Relative size also affects the relative perceived distance of two similarly shaped areas. In general, the larger area appears to be closer to the viewer than the smaller area (Ames, 1955; Ittelson, 1960). The proximal areas must be similar in shape, suggesting that they are treated as if they were the same object. Indeed, if it is assumed that they are the same object, then relative size perception is the same as perceptual constancy—the object must be nearer to produce the larger visual angle (see analysis of size perception in chapter 8).

Texture Gradient

Although a texture gradient is, strictly speaking, a pictorial cue to depth, it is a central conception in Gibson's (1950a) psychophysical approach. Consequently, the ideas surrounding texture and gradients are developed in detail in chapter 9. A brief description is presented here for completeness.

Surfaces have texture produced by the elements from which they are composed. The texture is represented in the light reflected from the surface. When a surface is viewed at a slant, the projected texture elements gradually change in size and shape over the projection surface. The changes follow the rules of perspective, i.e., the projected size decreases gradually for more and more distant parts of the distal surface. The projected shape of an element also changes gradually in perspective, depending on the position of the element.

Height in the Picture Plane

When the horizon is present in the visual field, objects whose proximal projection is close to the horizon appear to be farther from the viewer than objects whose proximal projection is farther from the horizon (Gibson, 1950a; see figure 9.4 for details). Clearly, the relationships implied by height–in–picture–plane apply only for a ground plane. They are reversed for a cloudy sky or the ceiling of a large room.

Rock, Shallo, and Schwartz (1978) questioned the efficacy of height–in–the–plane as a cue to depth. They used perceived size to index perceived distance and found essentially no effect of height–in–the–plane using a blank background field or one that contained a single horizontal line. Rock et al. (1978) concluded that height–in–the–plane must be a consequence of perceiving a ground plane in depth, not a determinant of it. That is, they proposed that an object is located at the distance where one of its contours intersects the ground plane, but only after perceiving a particular plane in depth.

Occlusion, Overlay, Interposition, or Superposition

When distal objects are arrayed in 3D, portions of more distant objects may be cut off from view by objects that are closer to the viewer. This situation produces a proximal pattern with overlap, a pattern described as *overlay, occlusion, interposition,* or *superposition.* Figure 7.3 shows a proximal occlusion pattern: Area *B* has continuous contours and area *A* has contours that intersect the contours of *B* at right angles. Viewers of this pattern report that area *B* appears closer than area *A* and that the common contour appears to belong to *B.* In general, when the outlines of two proximal objects intersect, the object whose contours are continuous at the point of intersection appears closer, and the common contour appears to belong to this object.

The operation of occlusion has been demonstrated on an apparatus that Ames (1955) called a *thereness-thatness table.* Figure 7.4 shows two arrays of cards in the two viewing alleys of the table. The field on the left contains three square cards at different positions in depth; card *A* is nearest to the

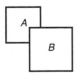

Figure 7.3
A simple occlusion pattern. Object *B* is closer to the viewer and obscures from view a portion of object *A.*

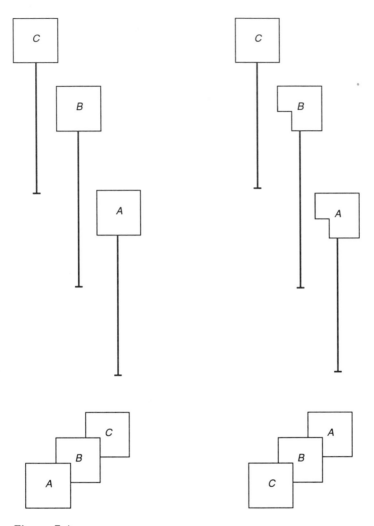

Figure 7.4
Two arrays of stimulus cards on the thereness–thatness table (Ames, 1955; Ittelson, 1952). The array on the left produces veridical perceived depth relationships and the one on the right produces inverse depth relationships.

viewer and card C is farthest from the viewer. The cards are aligned in such a way that a corner of the more distant card is occluded by the nearer card for an eye positioned at a specific point in space. The occlusion pattern produced in this way is shown below it: The contours of card A are continuous, and the contours of cards B and C change direction at the points of intersection. This proximal pattern is an occlusion pattern that results in the perception of three cards arrayed in depth in the same sequence as the real cards: A closer than B, closer than C. The surfaces of B and C appear to continue behind A and B, respectively.

The field on the right of figure 7.4 produces a similar proximal pattern. It is produced, however, in a very different way. In this case, the proximal area of card A in the original pattern is now produced by a card at the distance of card C. To accomplish this, a notch was cut in card B so that card B in the distal stimulus was exactly the same shape as area B in the proximal stimulus. Similarly, a notch was cut in card A so that card A in the distal stimulus was exactly the same shape as area A in the proximal stimulus. Thus, when viewed from the exact position that aligns the edges of the cards at the notches, this field of cards projects the same proximal stimulus as the left field, regardless of the actual distal stimulus configuration. Now card C appears to be the closest card and card A appears to be the most distant. Thus, with no additional information about the nature of the cards, the two fields of blank cards look identical.

Illumination and Reflectance Edges

Edges in the proximal stimulus can be produced in different ways. An edge produced entirely by illumination differences is called an *illumination edge*. This occurs, for example, when a uniform reflecting surface is illuminated by two different light sources, or when one surface occludes a portion of another surface making a shadow. An edge produced by two adjacent surfaces of different reflectances is called a *reflectance edge*. Obviously, illumination edges do not reflect properties of the distal world, whereas reflectance edges supply information about the surfaces of objects in space. Gilchrist (1977) showed that the 3D layout of space must be determined before lightness values can be assigned to surfaces.

Shading and Shadow

In most situations, distal objects reflect light from the sun or other light sources. The relative positions of the objects, the viewer, and the light source determine the differential pattern of light intensities reflected to the eye of the viewer. The directed nature of light produces both shading and shadow, which are different aspects of this pattern that carry potential information about relative depth, object shape, and the nature of the surfaces from which light is reflected. Therefore, both have been described as pictorial cues to depth and to object shape.

Shading describes differences in reflected flux, which are a consequence of variation in the angle between incident light and a surface. *Specular shading* describes the consequences of the light reflected from shiny surfaces, like that from a mirror. This type of shading is affected by the position of the observer and the direction of illumination. *Diffuse* or *Lambertian shading* describes the effects of light scattered in all directions as a consequence of reflection from a matte surface. The proximal pattern of shading produced in this case depends on how each local surface patch is oriented with respect to its sources of illumination (Norman & Todd, 1994). Thus, illumination edges may occur when surfaces of the same reflectance have different angles to the same single light source. There is also a more subtle aspect of shading, a self-masking in concavities. Surface concavities tend to receive less incident light because their geometry reduces the acceptance angle for diffuse light that is always present in the environment.

Shading can provide information about surface orientation. Gibson (1950a) suggested that shading can produce the perception of three-dimensionality in objects and scenes. He noted that a perceived scene is organized so that it appears to be illuminated by a single light source and, typically, the light appears to come from above. These organizing principles determine whether portions of the stimulus appear as protrusions or as depressions. The patterns illustrated in figure 7.5 demonstrate these principles (Ramachandran, 1988). The circular objects in (a) are shaded on the left or the right. Each object may appear to be either convex or concave, depending on the perceived direction of the light source falling on the object, and the viewer may reverse the perceived depth by consciously shifting the apparent light source.

It is clear, however, that the apparent change in perceived depth occurs simultaneously for the entire array, indicating that the perceived direction of light is applied globally over the entire array. The circles in (b) are shaded on either the upper or lower portion. These objects are usually organized spontaneously by the assumption that the light is overhead (Ramachandran,

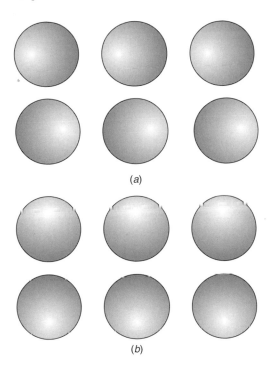

(a)

(b)

Figure 7.5
Effects of shading on relative perceived depth. Each object may appear to be convex
or concave depending on the perceived direction of the light source (Ramachandran, 1988).

1988), an assumption based primarily on retinal rather than gravitational
information (Kleffner & Ramachandran, 1992).

In experimental studies, shading has been found to be, at best, a weak
cue to shape. Many studies describe large differences in reports of perceived
shape among different viewers of the same stimuli (see Pollick, Watanabe,
& Kawato, 1996, for a review) and, in recent investigations (Erens, Kappers,
& Koenderink, 1993a, 1993b), viewers of pure-shading stimuli reported that
they did not look like pictures of anything. Using a different approach,
Koenderink, van Doorn, Christou, and Lappin (1996) varied shading para-
metrically. They systematically changed the location of the source of illumination on an object, producing changes in the shading of the object due
to variations in the local surface attitude and *vignetting,* the screening of the
extended source by the object itself. They measured pictorial relief for
pictures of a smooth solid object and found that different directions of

illumination led to systematic alterations in perceived pictorial relief. In addition, brighter parts of the stimulus were interpreted as nearer in pictorial space, both for global layout and for subsidiary relief. Koenderink et al. (1996) concluded that shading is an important source of information about shape.

A *shadow* is an area that is blocked from illumination. Thus, a real shadow is always darker than adjacent nonshadow regions. An object produces a *cast shadow* when its shadow falls on another surface. Cast shadows produce sharp proximal discontinuities of illumination that project the shape of the object profile onto adjacent surfaces. An *attached shadow* is produced when an object's shadow falls on itself—a self-shadow. The shape of the shadow carries information about the 3D scene. Its shape is determined by several factors: the direction of the light source, the shape of the object casting the shadow, the surface relief on which it falls, and the relative positions of the light source, the object, and the receiving surface (Cavanagh & Leclerc, 1989).

The contributions of shadow shape to the perception of object shape were studied by Cavanagh and Leclerc (1989). Their results suggested that the interpretation of shadows begins with the identification of acceptable shadow borders. Thus, shadows provide a subset of object contours and a hypothesis about occluded object regions. Shadow contours provide information about surface convexities and enclosed shadow regions provide information about concavities.

Aerial Perspective

Light is scattered by particles in the atmosphere. Light from a far object is scattered away from the line of sight and light from the sky (the sky light) is scattered into the line of sight. Consequently, when a viewer looks at a distant object, there is a reduction of contrast in the proximal representation of the object, depending on its distance from the viewer. In addition, distant objects are less vivid in color than near objects, are more bluish in appearance, and may appear to be blurred. These components of *aerial perspective* provide information about the relative distances of objects in a scene (see O'Shea, Blackburn, & Ono, 1994, for a review).

Contrast is a function of the distance from the object to the viewer and of the degree of clarity of the atmosphere. As O'Shea et al. (1994) point out, it is not necessary for the air to contain particles such as dust or pollutants for scattering to occur—scattering of light by air molecules (Rayliegh scattering) produces an appreciable reduction of contrast for far objects even in perfectly clean air. Consequently, they note that aerial perspective is not a development of the Industrial Age but has been available as a cue to depth throughout the course of evolution.

O'Shea et al. (1994) performed an experiment to see if contrast is sufficient as a pictorial cue. Their stimuli were square patches of different luminance presented in pairs on a flat screen. Contrast was altered by varying the background luminance. Results showed that the higher-contrast member of the stimulus pair appeared closer than the lower-contrast member. O'Shea et al. (1994) concluded that contrast is a pictorial cue to depth that acts by simulating aerial perspective.

Information from Oculomotor Adjustments

Information classified as *physiological cues* includes neural information about muscle movements that control the positions of the eyes and the refractive states of the lenses.

Accommodation and Convergence

The change in the focal length of the lens of the eye when fixation distance changes is called *accommodation*. Retinal blur is generally thought to be the stimulus for changes in the ciliary muscles that produce accommodative changes in the lens of the eye. The result is to reduce the blur and sharpen the image on the retina.

When no stimulus is present, accommodation and convergence return to an idiosyncratic resting or tonus position of about 1 to 2 meters (Leibowitz & Owens, 1978; Owens & Leibowitz, 1983). When one eye is closed, there is an inward shift in accommodation so that the closed eye tends to return to its *resting accommodative distance* or *dark focus* (Leibowitz, Henessy, & Owens, 1975). This change tends to draw the open eye inward by the same amount (Roscoe, 1979). Adaptation of accommodation and convergence is demonstrated in consistent aftereffects of prior viewing conditions (Ebenholtz, 1988, 1991; Ebenholtz & Zander, 1987; Schor, 1983).

Oculomotor processes may directly affect depth perception (Ebenholtz, 1983; Enright, 1989; Owens & Leibowitz, 1983; Post & Leibowitz, 1985; Roscoe, 1989). Perceived size and perceived distance changes are sometimes associated with changes in vergence and accommodation.

Reduction in apparent size that accompanies reduction in focal distance of the lens is described as *accommodative micropsia*. Reduction in the apparent dimensions of a scene that accompanies artificially induced increases in convergence is described as *convergence micropsia*. It is not clear, however, whether the physiological changes are causes or consequences. One way around this dilemma is to suggest that the neural signals that trigger accommodation and convergence responses enter into the causal sequence that determine the perception of distance and of size (see Enright, 1989; McCready, 1965; Roscoe, 1989, for reviews).

Gradient of Focus

When one is looking at a 3D scene, the images on the retina are poorly focused. The fixated point is represented in nearly perfect focus at the center of the fovea and the remainder of the scene is represented by increasingly blurred images of points at increasing distances. The most distant points are almost completely blurred. Pentland (1987) demonstrated that this *gradient of focus* supplies information about distance between the viewer and points in the scene. In one experiment, increasing blur in pictures of a scene was perceived as increasing distance and, in a second experiment, the perceived direction of rotation of an outline cube was controlled by the focal gradient.

Eye Elevation

Elevation of the eyes produces a shift in the resting position of convergence away from the viewer (Heuer & Owens, 1987), and there is a decrease in apparent size with increasing elevation (Heuer, Wischmeyer, Brüwer, & Römer, 1991). Eye elevation has entered into explanations of apparent distance, especially in relation to the moon illusion (Holway & Boring, 1940). The evidence for this effect of eye elevation will be discussed in chapter 8 when alternative explanations of the moon illusion are presented.

Automatic Organizing Processes

It is frequently noted that relationships within the structure of the stimulus configuration play a role in determining the perceptual outcome. The Gestalt psychologists (Koffka, 1935; Köhler, 1929; Wertheimer, 1912, 1923/1937) devised demonstrations of fundamental perceptual phenomena to emphasize this view. They proposed that the neural processes underlying perception organize themselves spontaneously according to specific laws or principles. The operation of these principles can be observed in figure-ground organization, the Gestalt laws, apparent motion, induced motion, and subjective contours.

Figure-Ground Organization

Figure-ground relationships are illustrated in figure 7.6. In figure 7.6a, the the stimulus patch *(A)* appears to be an object that is closer to the viewer than the background *(B)*. The object has sharp (clear) contours whereas the ground generally does not have boundaries. The same portion of the field, *(A)*, can become part of the ground if a second contour is included so that it encloses A as in Figure 7.6b. In this case, area *B* becomes a figure with a hole in it. Area *A* now appears to be a continuation of the background *(C)* seen through the hole in *B*. The contour now appears to be part of *B* and

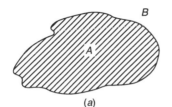

(a)

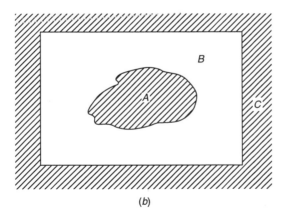

(b)

Figure 7.6
Figure-ground organization. (a) The figure *(A)* appears to be closer to the viewer than the ground *(B)* and the contour appears to belong to the figure. (b) These relationships can be reversed by adding a contour around *A*. Now *B* is the figure and *A* appears to be a hole through which the background is visible. The contour appears to be part of *B*.

the relative depth positions are reversed: *B* appears to be nearer to the viewer than *A* and *C*.

Cohen (1957) studied figure–ground relationships experimentally using a *Ganzfeld,* a homogeneous visual field. To produce the *Ganzfeld,* Cohen connected two spheres so that the interior of one sphere could be viewed through a circular opening. Each sphere was illuminated by a separate projector not visible to the viewer. When the illumination in the two spheres was the same, subjects reported seeing a contourless fog for a few moments and then reported that their visual experience ceased. When a small difference in illumination was introduced, the perceptual field appeared to be separated into a figure and a background. Thus, slight discontinuities in the visual field were represented by the visual system as an object in front of a ground.

Gestalt Organizational Laws

In the Gestalt account of perception various arrangements of stimulus elements are organized spontaneously in perception due to perceptual organizational processes. The Gestalt laws are the descriptive statements relating the characteristics in the stimulus to those in perception. Figure 7.7 illustrates some of these principles. The *law of proximity* is illustrated in fig-

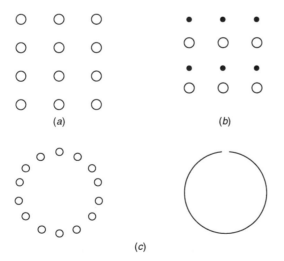

Figure 7.7
Some patterns illustrating the Gestalt laws. (a) *Proximity:* The dots appear to be arranged in columns. (b) *Similarity:* The dots appear to be arranged in rows. (c) *Closure:* The circles appear to be complete.

ure 7.7a for an array of similar elements. The elements are perceived as columns because the vertical separation between them is smaller than the horizontal separation. The *law of similarity* is illustrated in figure 7.7b for an array of equidistant dissimilar elements. This array is perceived as rows because the elements in the rows are similar. The *law of closure* is illustrated in figure 7.7c for a circle of elements and an almost complete circular line. Both appear to be complete circles, i.e., presumably, the visual system fills in the missing portions to complete the circles.

Figure 7.8 illustrates the *law of good continuation*. The pattern in the upper portion of the figure could be organized perceptually in two different ways. In terms of logical analysis, the two organizations illustrated in the lower portion of the figure are equally likely. However, viewers invariably report that the figure is perceived as a combination of the square and smooth-curve patterns. According to the Gestaltists, these patterns illustrate good continuation because they represent continuous repetition of simple geometrical patterns, i.e., they do not involve large angular changes in direction. *Common fate* adds the aspect of motion: Elements that move together tend to be grouped in perception (Wertheimer, 1923/1937). A similar relationship appears in Johansson's concept of common motion (chapter 12).

In the classical Gestalt view, "good" perceived patterns tend to be simple (Attneave, 1954, 1982) and ambiguous stimulus patterns tend to be organized into perceptions that can be described simply (Hochberg &

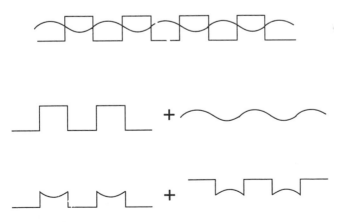

Figure 7.8
The law of *good continuation*. The figure may be logically organized in either of two ways but it is always perceived as illustrated in the middle figure.

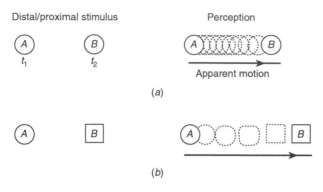

Figure 7.9
Apparent motion. (a) Light bulbs at positions A and B are flashed asynchronously (i.e., at t_1 and t_2, respectively). The perception is apparent motion of the light from A to B. (b) If the stimulus consists of objects of different shapes, the perceived moving object appears to change shape gradually as it moves.

McAlister, 1953; Hochberg & Brooks, 1960; Restle, 1982). These rules of perceptual organization have been described as a *minimum principle*. (See chapter 12 for Johansson's use of a minimum principle and Cutting & Proffitt, 1982, for a detailed discussion of the relations between the minimum principle and the perception of absolute, common, and relative motions.)

Apparent Motion
Wertheimer's (1912) analysis of *apparent motion* was an important milestone in the development of Gestalt psychology (and of motion perception; see Sekuler, 1996). The phenomenon is illustrated in figure 7.9a. Two lights, one at position A and one at B, are flashed in sequence: A at t_1 and B at t_2. With the appropriate temporal interval, A appears to move to B. There are two components to the perceptual experience: motion and object perception. The phenomenon is usually described as one of seeing motion when there is no motion in the stimulus. However, the second component is as important—the object appears to move in the area between the positions of A and B, an area of the visual field that received no stimulation.

Figure 7.9b illustrates the results of an experiment by Kolers (1972). If apparent motion is generated between two figures of different shapes, the shape appears to change gradually over the course of the motion from one to the other. A number of experiments have demonstrated that apparent motion is not determined by proximal stimulus variables but by the per-

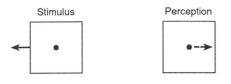

Figure 7.10
An illustration of induced motion (Duncker, 1929). Although the square frame actually moves to the left, it appears to remain stationary and the dot appears to move to the right.

ceived space in which the objects appear to move (Attneave & Block, 1973; Rock & Ebenholtz, 1962; Shepard & Judd, 1976).

Induced Motion

When a stationary object appears to move because of motion of some other object in the field, usually a surround, the motion of the stationary object is said to be *induced* (Duncker, 1929). Figure 7.10 shows a point surrounded by a rectangle. If the rectangle moves to the left, the rectangle appears stationary and the dot appears to move to the right. The perceived motion of the stationary dot is induced motion. Duncker (1929) suggested that the dot appears to move because the surrounding object serves as a frame of reference for the other object.

Duncker generalized induced motion to all object-relative motions by suggesting that, when there is a proximal distance change between two objects, one object serves as a frame of reference for the other (enclosed) object. This interpretation illustrates two rules of perceptual organization: First, the stimulus for perceived motion is relational and, second, perception is organized so that the surround (frame) is stable and the objects within it move. Mack, Heuer, Fendrich, Vilardi, and Chambers (1985) found that induced motion was accompanied by a shift in the judged direction of the straight-ahead and, therefore, was not based on oculomotor visual capture. This finding supports Duncker's object-relative explanation.

Subjective Contours

Occlusion and figure-ground relationships may be involved in the production of subjective or illusory contours (see Kanizsa, 1955; Lesher, 1995; Purghé & Coren, 1992, for reviews). In monocular vision, contours can appear to define a surface that fills unstimulated areas in the proximal stimulus just as they could in binocular vision. These *subjective contours* define

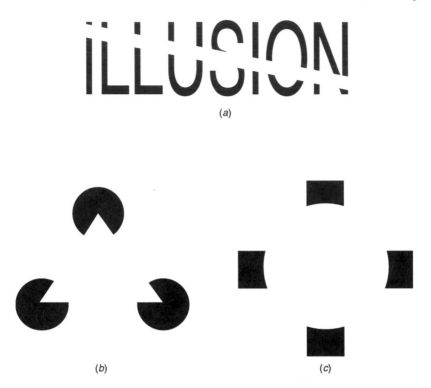

(a)

(b)   (c)

Figure 7.11
Subjective contours. (a) A bar appears to occlude a portion of the word *illusion;* (b) a triangle appears to occlude a portion of the circles; and (c) a circle appears to occlude a portion of the squares. The occluding objects appear to be surfaces with contours.

surfaces that play the same role as those in figure-ground. Figure 7.11 illustrates some stimuli that produce monocular subjective contours. In these examples, the contours appear to define an occluding surface that is closer to the viewer than other portions of the proximal pattern (Coren, 1972). This contour may be as complex as that needed to complete a word that is printed on a page.

Observer Tendencies

Gogel found that the perceived absolute distance of an object or the relative perceived distance between objects tends to approach certain specific values as depth information decreases. He described these mechanisms as *observer tendencies.* For example, a single object viewed monocularly in a dark room provides minimal perceptual input and appears to be localized at a distance of 2 to 4 meters (Gogel, 1969; Gogel & Da Silva, 1987a, 1987b; Gogel & Teitz, 1973). Gogel called this phenomenon the *specific distance tendency.*

The *equidistance tendency* refers to the perceived relative depth of two objects with nonoverlapping proximal projections. As the directional (angular) separation between the objects decreases, there is an increase in the tendency for the objects to appear equidistant from the viewer (Gogel, 1965, 1969). When the edges of the two objects coincide, the coincident edges will appear to be at the same distance from the viewer.

Summary

Monocular information in the proximal stimulus can be represented in a frontal plane projection, the *pictorial cues.* In linear perspective, the horizon is usually the boundary of a surface (the ground) that extends indefinitely into the distance. Parallel contours of receding surfaces project onto the frontal plane as converging lines that meet at vanishing points on the horizon. The separations between contours that are parallel to the frontal plane are compressed in the projection. For a perceiver on the ground, distant objects on the ground project higher in the proximal pattern than near objects. The shapes of the surfaces of distal objects project as perspective representations in the proximal pattern. Therefore, perspective in the proximal pattern supplies information about the relative depth of objects and of positions of objects in the field. The perspective information provided by surfaces at a slant is sometimes called outline shape. Thus, outline shape with perspective provides information for the perception of surface-at-a-slant. Other sources of information are shading and shadow, and aerial perspective.

Accommodation and convergence changes may also supply information about relative depth. Figure-ground organization, the Gestalt laws, and observer tendencies describe automatic organizing principles that govern monocular perceptions.

8

Empiricist View: Perceived Size and Shape

The classical empiricist analysis of perceived size and perceived shape is based on two invariance hypotheses: the size-distance invariance hypothesis (SDIH) and the shape-slant invariance hypothesis (SSIH). An entirely different approach to these problems—Gibson's psychophysical view—is described in the next chapter. A review of the vast literature on the topics contained in these two chapters can be found in Sedgwick (1986).

Perceived Size of Afterimages

The proximal stimulus produced by a distal object of size S at distance D from the observer was described in chapter 6: $\tan \alpha = S/D$. Recall that, in this distal-proximal relationship, *size* is a property of the object and *distance* refers to the space between the viewer and the object. Consequently, physical size and physical distance are independent quantities. In contrast, the corresponding quantities in the perceptual world, perceived size s and perceived distance d, are not independent; they are properties of perceptual experience. The discussion of perceived size and distance begins with afterimages. It describes Emmert's law of afterimage size and its use as a model for the perceived size of objects.

Emmert's Law of Afterimages

An *afterimage* is a visual image that is seen after the physical stimulus is removed. It may be formed by looking at a light or an illuminated object and then looking away at a surface. An image of the object or the light will be seen on the surface. The image has a definite size and shape, and appears to be at the same distance from the viewer as the surface upon which it is projected.

Figure 8.1 shows the simple relationships involved in viewing an afterimage. Figure 8.1a shows the adapting stimulus, e.g., a light of size S_L at a distance D_L from the viewer, that subtends a visual angle α: $\tan \alpha = S_L/D_L$. The viewer fixates the light for a few seconds and then looks at a gray wall. An image of the light appears on the wall, the afterimage.

Figure 8.1b shows the geometrical relationships involved in the perceived size of the afterimage. The wall is at an arbitrary distance, D', from the viewer. The perceived size of the afterimage that appears to be on the surface at D' is given by:

$$s = D' \tan \alpha. \tag{8.1}$$

Equation 8.1 is one possible formulation of Emmert's law: The perceived size of the afterimage varies directly with viewing distance (Emmert, 1881). However, D' is the physical distance of the surface, and physical quantities cannot enter mental processing to determine perception. This issue can be avoided by noting that the surface appears to be at the perceived distance d'. Therefore, the perceived size of the afterimage is given by:

$$s = d' \tan \alpha. \tag{8.2}$$

This is Emmert's law (see Hochberg, 1971, for a review of Emmert's law and constancy).

Registered Distance

In Equation 8.2, d' is a perceptual outcome, the perceived distance of the wall. Therefore, it cannot enter the causal sequence as a determiner of s, a simultaneous perceptual outcome. To solve this problem, some theorists have distinguished conceptually between perceived distance and registered distance (Epstein, 1973; Kaufman & Rock, 1962, 1989; Rock, 1975; Rock & Kaufman, 1962; Wallach & Berson, 1989; Wallach & Floor, 1971; Wallach & Frey, 1972). *Registered distance D,* describes stimulus information about distance that is encoded and, therefore, enters perceptual processing to affect perceptual outcomes. Registered distance can be distance information produced by any of the distance cues in the proximal stimulus or by oculomotor adjustments. Depending on the specific situation, registered distance information may or may not affect perceived size or perceived distance. For example, in Kaufman and Rock's (1962) explanation of the paradoxical size–distance relations in the moon illusion, registered distance determines perceived size but not perceived distance (see the section on the

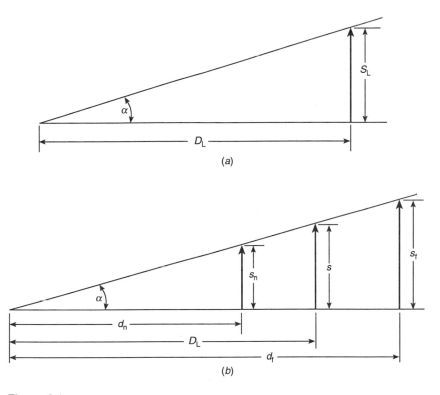

Figure 8.1
Emmert's law: the relationships involved in viewing an afterimage. (a) The adapting stimulus, a light of size S_L at distance D_L from the viewer, subtends a visual angle, α. (b) An afterimage of the light appears on a wall at distance D' from the viewer. If the wall appears to be more distant (d_f), the afterimage appears larger (s_f); if the wall appears closer (d_n), the afterimage appears smaller (s_n).

moon illusion, below). Obviously, registered distance is an inferred concept that remains controversial even among empiricists.

In the afterimage case, one could argue that information about the distance of the wall enters the processing sequence prior to the determination of the perceived size and distance of the afterimage. In this interpretation, registered distance determines perceived distance: $d = D_r$ and, in another formulation of Emmert's law, the perceived size of the afterimage is given by the algorithm:

$$s = D_r \tan \alpha. \tag{8.3}$$

Figure 8.1b illustrates the fact that an afterimage changes in perceived size as the information about the distance of the wall and, in this case, the perceived distance of the wall, changes. This relationship was demonstrated by Ames (Ittelson, 1968). An afterimage of size s was projected onto a card at a fixed distance D from the viewer. The card was made to appear closer to (d_n) or farther away from (d_f) the viewer by means of occlusion (see chapter 7). When the card appeared nearer $(d_n < D)$, the afterimage was smaller $(s_n < s)$ and, when the card appeared to be farther away $(d_f > D)$, the afterimage was larger $(s_f > s)$. Thus, the perceived size was not determined by the actual distance of the card. In this case, the relative distance information (registered distance) determined both the perceived size and the perceived distance of the afterimage. A similar change in the apparent size (Dwyer, Ashton, & Broerse, 1990) and shape (Broerse, Ashton, & Shaw, 1992) of an afterimage has been demonstrated using the distorted room (see below) to alter the apparent distance of the surface on which the afterimage was projected.

Thus, Emmert's law predicts that the size of an afterimage varies directly with the distance information about the surface on which it is projected. Consequently, afterimages have been used as a tool to investigate the perceived distance of surfaces. For example, King and Gruber (1962) had subjects form afterimages and project them onto the sky. They compared the relative size of the afterimages at different elevations to determine the relative perceived distance of the sky at each elevation. King and Gruber found that the size of the afterimage was largest at the horizon and smallest at zenith: $s_h > s_{(45\,\text{deg})} > s_z$. They inferred, therefore, that the perceived distance of the sky varies directly as the perceived size of the afterimage: $d_h > d_{(45\,\text{deg})} > d_z$. That is, they demonstrated experimentally that the sky is perceived as a flattened dome.

Hypotheses of Invariance

An *invariance hypothesis* defines the relationship between the proximal stimulus and perception. It is a refined notion of stimulus determinism. In general, invariance hypotheses state that, for a given proximal stimulus, the perception will be one of the distal configurations that could have produced that proximal pattern. Note that the definition does not state which of the possible distal configurations will be seen. Thus, an invariance hypothesis can be considered a rule or algorithm that relates aspects of perception to aspects of stimulation.

Size-Distance Invariance Hypothesis

Starting from an analysis of stationary objects, the traditional form of the *size-distance invariance hypothesis* describes the perceptions that are possible for a given constant visual angle (Epstein, 1977b; Epstein, Park, & Casey, 1961; Gilinsky, 1951; Ittelson, 1951a, 1951b, 1960; Kilpatrick & Ittelson, 1953; Oyama, 1977; Weintraub & Gardner, 1970). One formulation asserts that the ratio of perceived size to perceived distance is constant, i.e., perception is constrained by the proximal stimulus, in this case the the visual angle. Thus, a given visual angle α determines a ratio of perceived object size s to perceived object distance d:

$$s/d = \tan \alpha. \tag{8.4}$$

Note the difference between equations 8.3 and 8.4—this form of the SDIH is not Emmert's law.

Figure 8.2 illustrates three possible perceptions that satisfy equation 8.4: $s_1/d_1 = s_2/d_2 = s_3/d_3 = \tan \alpha$. Clearly, the SDIH does not constrain the absolute values of perceived size or perceived distance. It only constrains their ratio (s/d). Assuming the SDIH, s and d vary directly for a given visual angle: As perceived size s increases, perceived distance d increases, and vice versa. Obviously, in this formulation, additional information is required to combine with a given visual angle input in determining a unique perceptual outcome. With respect to size, additional information can come from the familiar or known size of a given stimulus, or from relative size when two

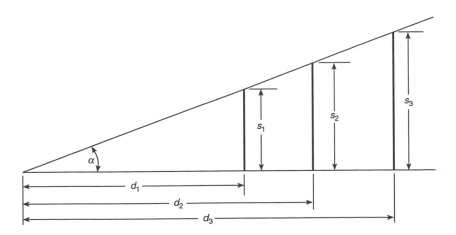

Figure 8.2
Three possible perceptions that satisfy equation 8.4: $s_1/d_1 = s_2/d_2 = s_3/d_3 = \tan \alpha$.

or more stimuli are present. With respect to distance, additional information can come from many different input sources, e.g., pictorial and oculomotor cues.

An alternative formulation of the SDIH (Kaufman & Rock, 1962, 1989; Rock, 1975; Rock & Kaufman, 1962; Wallach & Berson, 1989; Wallach & Floor, 1971; Wallach & Frey, 1972) holds that accurate size perceptions are determined by the Emmert's law algorithm, in which the perceived size of an object is determined by visual angle and registered distance. In this formulation, the invariance hypothesis relates perceived size to registered distance rather than to perceived distance. In a particular instance, perceived distance may or may not be affected by the same registered distance information that determines perceived size. When registered distance determines perceived distance, the perception is veridical and the SDIH holds as stated in Equation 8.3. However, when perceived distance is determined by factors other than the specific registered distance information that is producing the perceived size, the perceived-size–perceived-distance relations do not satisfy equation 8.3. Indeed, in some cases (e.g., the moon illusion), perceived size and perceived distance vary inversely.

Shape-Slant Invariance Hypothesis

Although the distal world contains solid objects, a viewer can see only the outer surfaces. These surfaces are extended in two dimensions and, therefore, subtend solid visual angles in the optic array. That is, the light reflected from a surface stimulates a retinal area. These spatial characteristics define the *shape* of a rigid object or surface. They do not change with translation, rotation, or change of scale.

The *shape-slant invariance hypothesis* asserts that a given proximal shape determines the possible perceived shapes at perceived slants (Beck & Gibson, 1955; Epstein, 1973; Koffka, 1935; Massaro, 1973). It is similar in form to the SDIH. A similar analysis can be applied to the SSIH, suggesting that additional information is required to specify a unique perceptual outcome. Thus, the perception of slant depends on information about shape, and the perception of shape depends on information about slant, or on psychological factors such as past experience, and Gestalt organizing mechanisms (Beck & Gibson, 1955; Epstein, 1977b; Epstein & Park, 1963; Flock, 1964a, 1964b; Koffka, 1935; Oyama, 1977). For example, Epstein (1973) proposed a "taking-into-account" hypothesis similar to that for the SDIH: Perceived shape is determined by a rule that takes slant into account in the processing of proximal projective shape. This formulation requires a registered slant concept similar to that of registered distance.

Perceived Size of Objects

The physical size of an object is described by the extent of its surfaces in 3D space. *Perceived size* is the quality of a perceived object that corresponds to its physical size.

Measuring Perceived Size: Brunswick and Thouless Ratios

The perceived size of a stationary object is frequently measured in experiments using a matching procedure. The *standard stimulus* is the object whose perceived size is being measured. The viewer adjusts the size of a similar object, the *variable* or *comparison stimulus,* until it appears to match the size of the standard. Typically, perceived size of an object is measured at different distances. Therefore, in experiments, the distance of the standard changes from measurement to measurement while the distance of the comparison does not.

The accuracy of the match can be assessed in different ways based on the assumption that the physical size of the comparison is an index of the perceived size of the standard. Under this assumption, the perceived and physical sizes of the standard can be compared directly. Because direct comparison has many shortcomings, Brunswick (1929) proposed an alternative formulation relating the matches to visual angle size. The *Brunswick ratio* (BR) relates the difference between the comparison and visual angle size to the difference between the standard and the visual angle size:

$$BR = (S_c - s_c)/(S - s_c), \tag{8.5}$$

where S_c is the size of the comparison, s_c is the visual angle or projected size of the standard at the distance of the comparison, and S is the physical size of the standard. Thouless (1931) proposed an alternative formulation that does not depend on which object is the standard and which is the comparison. This measure is called the *Thouless ratio* (TR):

$$TR = (\log S_c - \log s_c)/(\log S - \log s_c). \tag{8.6}$$

Both ratios vary between 0.0 and 1.0, where zero indicates a match to the visual angle subtended by the standard and 1.0 indicates a perfect match to its real size, or size constancy (see Myers, 1980, and Sedgwick, 1986, for detailed discussions).

Size Constancy

Despite the fact that a rigid object subtends different visual angles when it is viewed at different distances, its perceived size does not change. This aspect of stability in the perception of objects in space is described as *size constancy* (Epstein, 1977b; Epstein, Park, & Casey, 1961).

Holway and Boring (1941) demonstrated this basic fact of perception in an experiment that measured the effect of distance information on matched size. Subjects viewed stimulus discs of different sizes that were at different distances down a long corridor (10 to 120 feet), but always subtended the same visual angle (1 deg). They matched the perceived size of the discs using an adjustable disc of light in an intersecting corridor 10 feet away. When the stimuli were viewed either binocularly or monocularly with full distance information, the matches approximated size constancy values. When the depth information was decreased by viewing through an aperture that reduced the distance cues (a *reduction screen*), the size matches were greatly reduced. When the depth information was further reduced, the matches approached visual angle size.

One explanation for size constancy describes the perceptual processing as "taking distance into account" (Epstein, 1973, 1977b; Rock, 1975, 1977; Wallach & Floor, 1971; Wallach & Frey, 1972). In this view, registered distance information, the distance information available in everyday stimulation, is used in the processing to determine perceived size. With distance information given, the SDIH takes the form of equation 8.3 and perceived size is determined. The thereness-thatness table described in figure 7.4 illustrates how distance information can determine perceived size. In the righthand field, the occlusion pattern produces reversal of the perceived distances for the near and far cards: The near card appears to be far away and, therefore, looks unusually large, whereas the far card appears to be near and, therefore, looks very small.

Leibowitz (1974) proposed that a number of different mechanisms (e.g., oculomotor adjustments, perceptual learning, and cognitive or conceptual processes) can contribute to determining size perception and size constancy. Leibowitz noted, for example, that size constancy matches for stimuli up to 1 meter away were predicted by values of accommodation and convergence (Leibowitz & Moore, 1966; Leibowitz, Shiina, & Hennessy, 1972). Beyond that distance, constancy was underestimated. Furthermore, Harvey and Leibowitz (1967) found that eliminating visual distance cues by a reduction screen did not affect size judgments at distances less than 1 meter.

Leibowitz also noted that size matches are affected by instructions (Carlson, 1960, 1977; Gilinsky, 1955, 1989; Leibowitz & Harvey, 1967, 1969). For example, Gilinsky (1955) presented triangles of different sizes (42 to 78 inches) outdoors at different distances between 100 and 4,000 feet. A matching stimulus was placed at 100 feet, 36 deg to the right. *Objective* instructions asked subjects to match the size of the test stimulus as if it were placed beside the matching stimulus. That is, they were to match how big the triangle "really is." *Picture image* instructions asked subjects to imagine looking at a picture and to match the size of the portion of the picture that would be cut off by the stimulus. The objective or "true size" instructions yielded a slight overestimation *(overconstancy)* over the entire range (see Teghtsoonian, 1974, for a discussion of this issue). The picture image instruction yielded matches that approached visual angle. In a subsequent study, more specific visual angle instructions produced a closer match to visual angle for targets places at 10 to 100 feet (Gilinsky, 1989).

Familiar Size

In addition to visual angle, size information is frequently available as *familiar* or *known size* (Ames, 1955; Ittelson, 1960). If the object is familiar and has a known size *(s_f)*, the SDIH becomes:

$$d = s_f/\tan \alpha, \tag{8.7}$$

and perceived distance is determined. Figure 8.3 illustrates the operation of familiar size. A normal sized playing card, S_N, is photographed and enlarged to size S_L. The enlarged card is placed at distance D and subtends the same visual angle as the normal card for a viewer at P. The card is viewed in a dark room, so there is no additional information about its size or distance. The viewer reports seeing a normal sized playing card *(s = S_N)* at a distance d that satisfies the SDIH. Thus, in this situation, familiar size and visual angle determine perceived distance.

Gogel questioned the role of familiar size based on studies in which two different responses were used to index perceived distance (Gogel, 1977, 1981). One measure was simple verbal report. The other was a procedure in which the head was moved laterally so that motion parallax (see

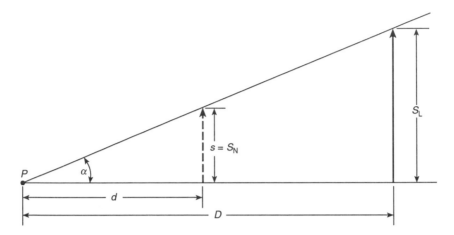

Figure 8.3
Familiar size. A normal sized playing card, S_N, is photographed and enlarged to size S_L. The enlarged card is placed at a distance, D. The viewer reports seeing a normal sized playing card ($s = S_N$) at a distance, d.

chapter 10) provided information about relative depth. Gogel found that the verbal reports of perceived distance increased as a function of familiar size whereas head-motion measurements were unchanged. Gogel suggested that perceived distance did not change in the experiment. He concluded, therefore, that the verbal reports represented the influence of cognitive factors (Gogel & Da Silva, 1987a). The role of familiarity is further complicated by Predebon's (1991) finding that, although familiar size influenced the relative egocentric distance of objects, it did not affect judgments of exocentric extents at distances from 5 to 80 meters. Predebon agreed with Gogel's assessment that nonperceptual (cognitive) factors influenced the distance reports.

Perceived Visual Angle

When distance information is not available, as, for example, when a luminous object is viewed in the dark, viewers can match the visual angle fairly accurately (Epstein & Landauer, 1969; Hastorf & Way, 1952; Lichten & Lurie, 1950; Rock & McDermott, 1964). This ability suggests that there are two types of size perceptions: object or linear size and extensivity or visual angle size (Rock, 1975, 1977; Rock & McDermott, 1964). *Visual angle size,* or the proportion of the visual field that the object subtends, is not normally in our awareness and is seldom brought into awareness without effort.

McCready (1965, 1985, 1986) noted that perceived visual angle α' is usually assumed to be equal to the actual visual angle: $\alpha' = \alpha$. In this view, linear and angular size responses are treated as two ways of measuring the same perceptual experience. Furthermore, perceived size and perceived distance are affected by visual cues, while perceived visual angle is treated as a direct response to retinal size.

McCready proposed a different conception of visual angle size. He defined *visual angle* as the optical direction difference between the edges of an object and *perceived visual angle size,* α', as the difference between the corresponding perceived directions. Furthermore, he assumed that the experiences associated with linear size and angular size are qualitatively different but simultaneously existing perceptual experiences. Thus, in his conception, when stimulated by an object of size S at distance D subtending a visual angle α, the object has a perceived linear size s at perceived distance d, and simultaneously, the object subtends a perceived visual angle α'.

In McCready's formulation of the SDIH, the two types of perceived size are not interchangeable. They are related according to a new SDIH:

$$s/d = \alpha'. \tag{8.8}$$

Thus, for McCready, the perceived-size–perceived-distance ratio is an invariant function of the perceived visual angle, not of the visual angle normally used to describe the proximal stimulus. Consequently, perceived visual angle has a unique status in the processing sequence and the two visual angles are related:

$$\alpha' = m(R/n) = m\alpha, \tag{8.9}$$

where R is the retinal extent of stimulation, n is the distance from the retina to the nodal point of the eye, and m is the phenomenal magnification, the ratio of perceived to actual visual angle.

Perceived Distance in a Scene

The perceived distance from the viewer to an object is called *egocentric distance* and the perceived distance between objects in the field is called *exocentric distance*. The perceived distances in a scene have been measured in many ways, including absolute estimates, map drawings, and comparisons among triad distances. Generally, these measurements produce a linear relationship between physical distance and judged distance up to 30 meters or so, a relationship that holds for both egocentric and exocentric distances

(Gilinsky, 1951; Levin & Haber, 1993; Toye, 1986; Wagner, 1985; Wiest & Bell, 1985).

Accurate judgments of distance have also been reported for distances between 30 and 100 meters (Gilinsky, 1989; Haber, 1983). Thus, perceived distance corresponds fairly well to real distance up to about 100 meters. Levin and Haber (1993) found a slight difference between estimates of distances oriented closer to the line of sight and those oriented closer to the frontal plane. The perceived distance between objects was slightly distorted as a function of the angular separation between objects. This resulted in an overestimation of distance in the frontal plane, which made the scene appear slightly elliptical along the horizontal axis. Consequently, perceived distances in the scene changed when the viewer changed position.

Perceived Shape of Objects

Perceived shape is the quality of a perceived object that corresponds to its physical shape.

Shape Constancy

Despite the fact that the proximal projection of a rigid object has different shapes when it is at different slants with respect to the viewer, the object appears to retain its shape. This phenomenon is described as *shape constancy*. In empiricist theory, shape constancy is a special case of the *shape-slant invariance hypothesis* (Beck & Gibson, 1955; Epstein, 1973; Epstein & Park, 1963; Koffka, 1935; Massaro, 1973; Pizlo, 1994; Sedgwick, 1986). Because the SSIH only determines a family of equivalent shapes at different slants, additional information is necessary for shape constancy to occur. This can be visual information about the shape of the object or the slant (orientation) of the surface, or cognitive information about the object's shape.

Familiar Shape

One source is familiarity with the shape of an object. The operation of this kind of information is illustrated in figure 8.4 for a trapezoidal window (Ittelson, 1968). The window is constructed as illustrated in figure 8.4a, which shows a perspective view of a real rectangular window *(C, D, E, F)* in the frontal plane of a viewer at point *P*. The window is projected onto an imaginary plane rotated about the axis *AB* so that it is slanted with respect to the viewer. In the slanted plane, the window will be trapezoidal in shape.

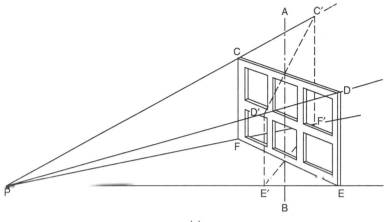

(a)

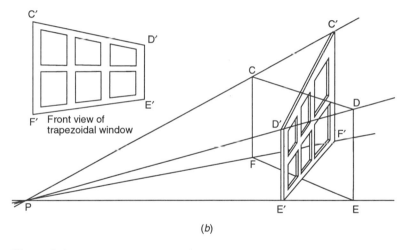

(b)

Figure 8.4
Construction of a trapezoidal window. (a) Real rectangular window *CDEF* is projected onto a plane at a slant producing trapezoidal window *C'D'E'F'*. The trapezoidal window is then constructed from a rigid material. (b) The trapezoidal window appears to be a rectangular window at a different slant.

Figure 8.4b shows the trapezoidal window C', D', E', F'. If this window is made into a real cardboard, wood, or metal window placed Cn appropriate slant to a viewer at point P, it appears to be a rectangular window in the frontal plane. If the trapezoidal window were placed C different slant, the rectangular window would appear to be C slant. According to Ames (Ittelson, 1968), the window appears rectangular because our past experience with windows has been predominantly with rectangular windows. That is, our familiarity with the shape of the object determines its perceived shape, and the SSIH determines its perceived slant.

Distorted Room

Both SDIH and SSIH relationships are involved in the *distorted room,* another of the Ames demonstrations (Ames, 1955; Ittelson, 1968). Figure 8.5 shows how the rear wall of a distorted room is constructed. A front view of a real rectangular room with two rectangular windows in the rear wall *(ABCD)* is shown on the right side of the figure. The left side of the figure shows a top view of the rear wall viewed from point P. This wall is projected onto an imaginary plane at a slant to the wall. Side AD projects to $A'D'$ and side BC projects to $B'C'$. Because the imaginary plane is at a slant to the real wall, the rectangular shapes project in perspective as trapezoids. Trapezoidal projections of the side walls, floor, and ceiling are obtained in the same way.

The projections are made into real objects from material such as plywood and painted to look like the original room. Figure 8.6 illustrates the situation when a viewer places an eye at P and looks into the trapezoidal room (solid lines in the figure). The room appears to be rectangular (dashed lines in the figure). The other parts of the trapezoidal room (windows, floor and ceiling patterns) also appear to be rectangular and to fit appropriately into the perceived room. In the transactionalist view, the unique perception is determined by our past experience with rectangular environments and the SSIH (Ames, 1955; Ittelson, 1968). The walls appear rectangular and, combined with the SSIH, the slant of the rear wall is determined (in this case a frontal plane).

Figure 8.7 shows two women of approximately the same size in opposite corners of the room. One woman looks very large and the other looks very small. A number of factors enter into this perceptual outcome. In reality, the woman on the right is nearer to the viewer and the woman on the left is farther away from the viewer. Therefore, the woman on the left subtends a smaller visual angle than the woman on the right. The

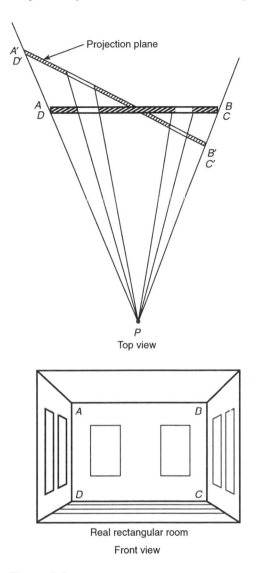

Figure 8.5

Construction of the rear wall of a distorted room (Ames, 1955; Ittelson, 1968). The bottom of the figure shows a front view of a real rectangular room with two rectangular windows in the rear wall, *(ABCD)*. The top shows a top view of this wall and its projection onto an imaginary plane at a slant to the wall. Side *AD* projects to *A'D'* and side *BC* projects to *B'C'*. Because the imaginary plane is at a slant to the real wall, the rectangular shapes project in perspective as trapezoids.

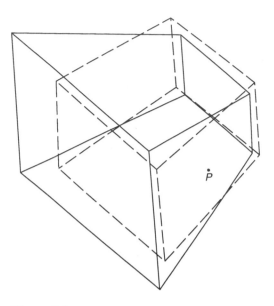

Figure 8.6
A distorted room (solid lines) viewed from point P appears to be a rectangular room
(dashed lines).

women occlude a portion of the rear wall and, therefore, appear to be in
front of it (i.e., closer to the viewer than the wall). Furthermore, the
women's feet are approximately the same height in the picture plane, i.e.,
they intercept the floor at approximately the same vertical position (see
chapter 9 for a discussion of this information). Therefore, they appear to be
in front of the rear wall but close to it. The wall, however, appears to be
in a frontal plane. Therefore, the women appear to be at approximately the
same distance from the viewer.

This situation is illustrated in figure 8.8 with (a) a top view, (b) a side
view of the woman on the left, and (c) a side view of the woman on the
right. There is relative size information about the woman at the far end
$(A'D')$ because she is physically smaller than the surrounding corner. Because the wall appears closer than it is, she appears closer and, consequently
(following the the SDIH), appears even smaller. Similarly, there is relative
size information about the woman at the near end $(B'C')$. She is almost as
large as the surrounding area of the walls and even may touch the ceiling.
Because this portion of the wall appears to be farther away than it really is,
this woman also appears to be farther away. Consequently (following the
SDIH) she appears to be even larger, i.e., she looks like a giant.

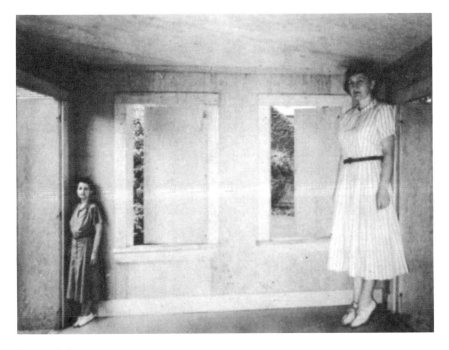

Figure 8.7
Perceptual outcome when two women of similar size stand in the corners of the distorted room. One woman looks very large and the other looks very small (Ittelson, 1968).

Noninvariance Perceptions

Despite many demonstrations where invariance formulations hold, the transactionalists (e.g., Ames, 1955; Ittelson, 1960) argued that perception is not limited to invariance outcomes. They suggested that perceptions can occur which do not satisfy invariance algorithms. The S-motion demonstration illustrates perceptions of size and distance that do not satisfy the SDIH.

S-Motion Demonstration

In the S-motion demonstration, perceived space was distorted using a trapezoidal window as illustrated in figure 8.4. Figure 8.9(a) shows a perspective view of the S-motion demonstration and figure 8.9(b) shows the arrangement from the top. Figure 8.10 shows a perspective view of the illusory motion. A trapezoidal window *(A'B')* was placed at a slant to the viewer and appeared to be a rectangular window *(AB)* at a different slant

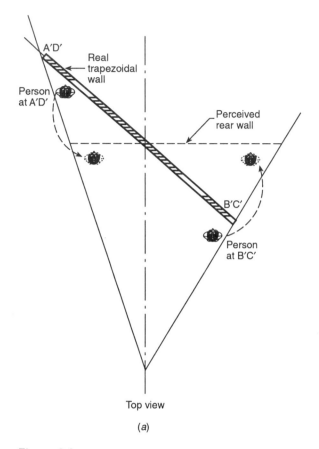

Top view

(a)

Figure 8.8
In the distorted room, one woman is nearer to the viewer at one end and the other is farther away from the viewer at the other end. However, they appear to be at approximately the same distance from the viewer. The top view of this situation is illustrated in (a). Side views are illustrated in (b) and (c).

to the viewer. The far end of the real trapezoidal window appeared to be the near end of the rectangular window and vice versa. A string passed though the righthand opening in the window and crossed the field in a frontal plane. A playing card mounted on the string moved through the window in the frontal plane. Therefore, the visual angle subtended by the playing card did not change as it moved because it was always in the frontal plane.

As the card moved across the visual field, it passed behind one side of the trapezoidal window and in front of the rest of the window. When it

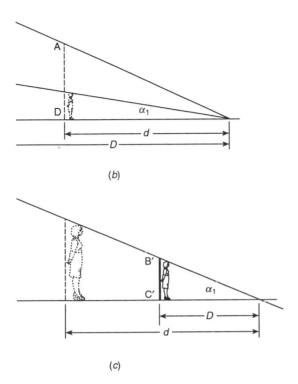

(b)

(c)

passed behind the window, the card was occluded, and, when it passed in front of the window, the card occluded portions of the window. This occlusion information determined the relative perceived depth of the card and window. But the trapezoidal window appeared to be in a plane whose slant was opposite that of the perceived rectangular window. Therefore, the card appeared to move in depth in an apparent "S" motion as it traversed the field (dotted line in the figure).

Viewers described the perceived size of this card as it moved in depth. The SDIH predicts that the card should appear smaller as it appears to move closer and larger as it appears to move away. However, viewers of the demonstration did not produce consistent reports (Ames, 1955; Ittelson, 1968). All possible combinations of perceived size and perceived distance changes were reported; there were also reports of no change in size. Ames concluded that size–distance perceptions are not limited by the SDIH, i.e., noninvariance perceptions are possible.

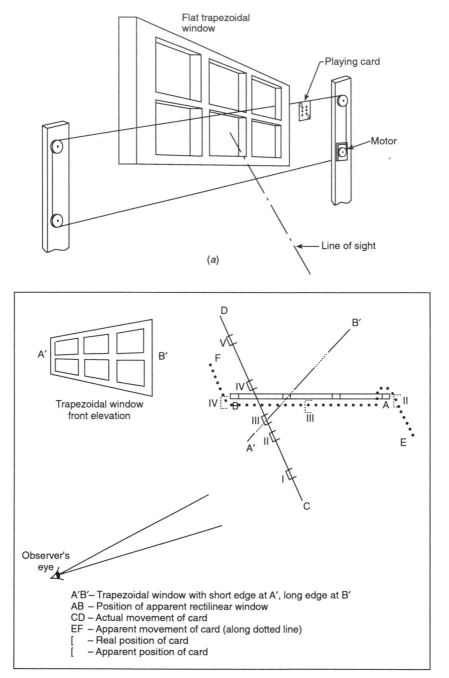

(a)

A′B′ – Trapezoidal window with short edge at A′, long edge at B′
AB – Position of apparent rectilinear window
CD – Actual movement of card
EF – Apparent movement of card (along dotted line)
[– Real position of card
[– Apparent position of card

(b)

Moon Illusion

The moon illusion may be a natural example of a common perceptual experience that does not follow the SDIH (Hershenson, 1982, 1989b). However, there is little agreement about the nature of the illusion despite the fact that it is one of the earliest known illusions. A reference to the illusion is clearly identifiable on clay tablets written as early as the seventh century B.C., and it was discussed by Aristotle, Ptolemy, and Ibn al-Haytham (Alhazan) among other early scientists (Plug & Ross, 1989). Thus, the illusion has been studied for over two millennia, yet it remains the subject of heated controversy (Hershenson, 1989a).

The visual angle stimulus produced by the moon does not change with elevation, i.e., there is no difference in the size of its image in a photograph of the moon at different elevations (see Solhkhah & Orbach, 1969, for a time-lapse photograph of the moon at different elevations). Nevertheless, the moon looks larger when it is near the horizon than when it is high in the sky (at zenith). There is no disagreement about this aspect of the illusion. The change in the perceived size of the moon as a function of elevation is the traditional description of the *moon illusion* and has been well documented (Plug & Ross, 1989). Similar illusions are produced by other objects in the sky. A sun illusion is easily observable at sunset and a celestial illusion that relates to other objects (e.g., stars, planets) and spaces (e.g., between stars) can be observed in the night sky (Hershenson, 1989a; Plug & Ross, 1989).

Indeed, the difficulty in finding an adequate explanation may be a consequence of another aspect of the illusion. Most observers report that the moon appears closer when it is near the horizon, and more distant when it is at zenith. This perceived-size–perceived-distance relationship contradicts the SDIH, revealing a *size-distance paradox* (Gruber, 1954; Hershenson, 1982, 1989a).

Many explanations have been offered for the moon illusion over the course of its long history (Plug & Ross, 1989). The most popular explanation in the first half of the twentieth century was based on eye elevation (Schur, 1925). She demonstrated that viewing an object in a dark room with eyes elevated made it appear smaller than when the eyes were horizon-

Figure 8.9
S-motion demonstration (a) in perspective and (b) from the top. A playing card moves across the field in a frontal plane. As it passes behind one part of the window and in front of the other part, the card appears to follow an S-shaped path (Ames, 1955; Ittelson, 1968).

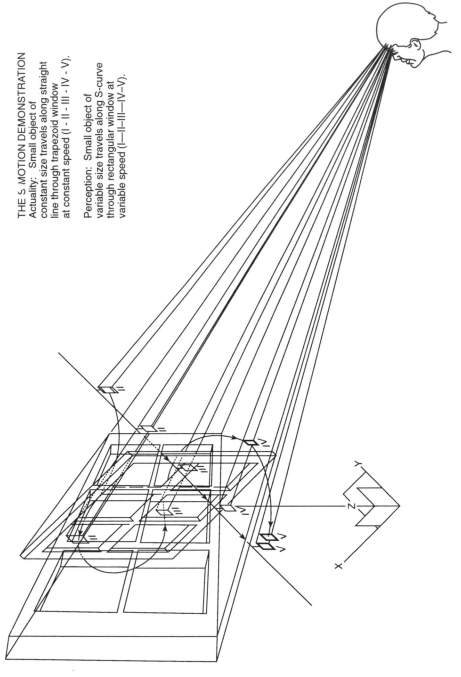

THE S MOTION DEMONSTRATION
Actuality: Small object of constant size travels along straight line through trapezoid window at constant speed (I - II - III - IV - V).

Perception: Small object of variable size travels along S-curve through rectangular window at variable speed (I—II—III—IV–V).

Figure 8.10
The S-motion demonstration in perspective (Ittelson, 1968). The playing card appears to travel around the window altering its distance from the viewer (see text for details).

tal. Taylor and Boring (1942) demonstrated a similar effect for direct observations of the moon. However, Kaufman and Rock (1962; Rock & Kaufman, 1962) tested the eye elevation hypothesis directly using a device that permitted viewing a moonlike object over a large expanse of ground or water with the eyes in various positions. They found no effect of eye elevation. Instead, they found that the horizon and surface terrain were the most important factors in the moon illusion.

Rock and Kaufman (1962) proposed a three-step explanation to incorporate their new finding: The terrain and horizon provide distance information that makes the area enclosed by the dome of the sky appear to be more distant at the horizon. This registered distance information enters the processing sequence in conjunction with the equidistance tendency to affect the perceived size of the moon. As the moon rises in the sky, the angular separation between the moon and the horizon becomes larger and larger. This change progressively weakens the effect of the equidistance tendency and provides information that the moon is getting closer and closer to the viewer.

In conjunction with the SDIH, this information results in a large perceived size for the moon at the horizon because of the great registered distance of the horizon. With increasing elevation, the decreasing registered distance produces a smaller perceived size of the moon. Rock and Kaufman (1962) suggested further that the reported distance of the moon is a consequence of cognitive analysis: The viewer reasons that the horizon moon looks large, large things are closer, therefore, the horizon moon must be closer. Notice that, in this explanation, registered distance determines perceived size but not perceived (reported) distance.

Gogel and Mertz (1989) proposed one of the few explanations of the paradox that retains the traditional formulation of the SDIH as a ratio of perceived size to perceived distance. They added a cognitive processing step between perception and the verbal response. In their view, relative perceived distance is determined by egocentric reference distance as a consequence of the specific distance tendency, the equidistance tendency, and oculomotor resting states. The equidistance tendency and the SDIH produce the greater perceived size and distance of the moon at the horizon. However, verbal descriptions of the moon's distance are determined by cognitive processes that produce a verbal report that the moon is close.

An entirely different explanation has been proposed by Hershenson (1982, 1989b). He agreed that the equidistance tendency interacts with the input distance information from the ground and horizon. However, instead of the SDIH (a static algorithm), Hershenson (1982) suggested that the mechanism operating in the moon illusion is a kinetic version of the invariance hypothesis (see chapter 11). This algorithm relates a changing visual angle to a constant perceived size for an object moving in depth. When presented with an object subtending the same visual angle at different perceived distances, this mechanism produces the moon illusion directly: a large perceived size for near objects and a small perceived size for far objects.

Summary

This chapter analyzed perceived size and shape from an empiricist point of view. The stimulus was described as a retinal extent (visual angle) or an outline shape, respectively. In this view, the stimulus is inadequate and cannot determine a unique percept. It must be supplemented by additional information from the stimulus or by cognitive (intelligent) processes such as inference, assumptions, or problem solving.

The possible perceptual outcomes may be constrained by various hypotheses of invariance. The SDIH constrains the ratio of perceived size and perceived distance to proximal stimulus size (visual angle). The SSIH constrains the perceived shape and perceived slant to the solid visual angle subtense. The demonstration of noninvariance perceptions, as in the S-motion demonstration and moon illusion, suggests that the invariance relationships may not be laws of perception but algorithms that work in most situations.

Gibson's Psychophysics—Basic Concepts

Gibson (1950a, 1959, 1966, 1979) argued that the traditional analysis of physiological optics resulted in a level of abstraction that lost much of the optical information. Instead of analyzing light rays and point stimulation, Gibson described the information in the total ambient optic array, an approach he called *ecological optics*. He described the optic array as a "super-stimulus" containing an abundance of redundant information about space. Gibson concluded that the stimulus appears to be inadequate in the traditional view only because it is analyzed into small units. When described in terms of the higher-order variables of ecological optics, visual stimulation is not inadequate. Consequently, perception is a direct response to information in the stimulus.

The central conception of ecological optics is the *ambient optic array,* the light surrounding an observer's position in the environment. This light is structured, but its structure must be considered from the point of observation, the position in space where a viewer might be and from which an act could be performed. Thus, while the abstract space of physiological optics consists of points and light rays, the space of ecological optics consists of places, locations, or positions that contain information about the layout of space as well as about the movement of the observer. This does not mean that the optic array is a qualitatively different abstract space, however. The difference is simply that the analysis of physiological optics reaches a greater level of abstraction of the same optical information.

The environment that provides this information is divided naturally into earth and sky, with objects on the earth and in the sky, and with some objects nested within others. All of these components contribute to the structure in the light at different observation points. Thus, the ambient optic array consists of a hierarchy of solid visual angles produced by the nested components of the environment at a common point of observation. The theoretical impact of Gibson's analysis of stimulation is that it permits identification of stimulus variables that determine aspects of perception directly, i.e., without the need for additional input from cognitive or experiential processes. Consequently, Gibson's view represents not only a different conception of stimulation, but a different understanding of its relation to the resulting perceptual experience.

Psychophysical Correspondence

In Gibson's formulation, understanding visual space perception requires identification of higher-order variables in stimulation that correlate with complex perceptual responses. If this can be accomplished, it is not necessary to invoke inference, past experience, learning, assumptions, guesses, or other cognitive processes to supplement input. This is Gibson's hypothesis of *psychophysical correspondence:* For every aspect or property of the phenomenal world there is a variable of the energy flux at the receptors, however complex, with which the phenomenal property would correspond if a psychophysical experiment could be performed.

Gibson argued that the visual field is invariably divided by a horizon into sky and ground. The sky supplies little information, but the horizon and ground (an extended surface) supply a lot of information about depth. One reason for this is that the eye is always in a head attached to a body that is (usually) standing on the ground. Thus, the eye is almost always above the ground. Because the horizon and ground were universally present during evolution, the relationship of eye to ground must have played an important role in the evolution of the eye-brain system. Therefore, Gibson's theory is a "ground" theory or an *eye-ground theory.*

Figure 9.1 illustrates one difference in Gibson's approach to the problem of distance perception. In the classical (empiricist) interpretation, distal points A, B, C, and D are aligned. Although the points are at different distal distances, they stimulate the same proximal point. Therefore, the proximal representation of the points does not contain information about the relative distance of the points. That is why the stimulus is inadequate. In contrast, a ground theory analysis treats the points as being embedded in a ground surface $(A'$, B', C', and $D')$. When stimulating an eye above the ground, the respective distal points are represented by different proximal points and

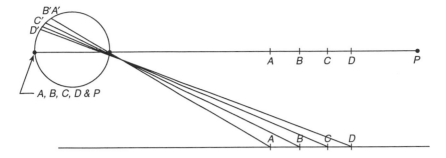

Figure 9.1
In classical analysis, distal points *A*, *B*, *C*, and *D* are aligned on the optic axis and stimulate the same proximal point. In Gibson's analysis, the points are embedded in a ground surface so that they are represented by different proximal points *(A', B', C'*, and *D')*.

the spaces between them are represented by gradually decreasing proximal distances. This proximal array carries distance information.

Texture and Optical Texture Gradient

Gibson began his analysis by describing a world that consists of objects and the ground on which the viewer stands. Although these are solid (3D) objects, the light that reaches the eye is primarily reflected from the surfaces of both objects and ground. Therefore, it is necessary to analyze the higher-order patterns in the projection of the optic array reflected from surfaces.

Texture
All real surfaces have a microstructure consisting of units that are relatively homogeneous in size, shape, and spacing over the surface. The surface quality produced by the microstructure is its *texture*. Different substances have different textures. For a given surface, the elements of texture may vary slightly so that they are the same only on average. Textures can also differ in *density*, the number of texture elements per unit surface area.

Optical Texture
The light reflected from distal surfaces retains the characteristics of the units in the surface, i.e., the light contains *optical texture*. The distal elements may be large or small, and the corresponding optical texture may be described

as coarse or fine. Surfaces may be at different distances from a viewer and, therefore, near surfaces may occlude more distant surfaces. Indeed, many surfaces may occlude many other surfaces. Therefore, the visible field of a viewer will contain a nested hierarchy of optical textures that can be analyzed in terms of the microstructure of surfaces (Gibson, 1950b, 1979).

By definition, the units of texture in a distal surface are approximately the same size and shape. If the surface is oriented in the frontal plane, the optical texture units in the picture plane are approximately the same size and shape. The density of the optical texture produced by the surface varies as a function of distance from the viewer. The relationship is illustrated in figure 9.2, which shows two surfaces containing the same textures at two different distances from a viewer (egocentric distance). The optical texture produced by the surface when viewed from the far position is compressed equally in all directions compared to the optical texture viewed from the

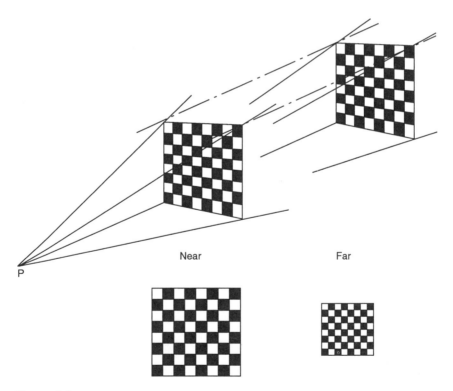

Figure 9.2
For a given textured surface, the density of *optical texture* varies as a function of viewing distance.

near position. The far surface has a greater optical texture density—there are more units of texture per unit area (solid visual angle) for the far surface than for the near surface.

When the eye is above the ground, however, the ground is a surface that is slanting away from the viewer. This slanting surface projects onto a picture plane with a gradual and continuous change in the size and shape of the units of optical texture. This gradual change in the optical texture is an *optical texture gradient*. The gradient is produced by two components: The texture units are progressively compressed (as in figure 9.2) due to the differences in their respective distances, and the vertical dimensions (altitudes) of the units are progressively foreshortened in the proximal stimulus due to the slant of the distal surface.

Figures 9.3 and 9.4 illustrate the optical texture gradient produced by a ground plane. Figure 9.3 shows a perspective view of a ground surface at a slant to a viewer at *P*. The distal surface contains square units that are projected onto a frontal plane to illustrate their representation in the proximal stimulus. Figure 9.4 shows top, side, and picture plane views of these relationships. Sides *A, B, C,* and *D* of the square texture elements run parallel to the frontal plane. The nearest *(D)* is represented lowest in the plane, and the most distant *(A)* is represented highest in the plane. Their proximal size decreases proportionally with distance from the eye.

The depth dimensions of the square texture elements *(a, b, c)* run perpendicular to the frontal plane. The nearest *(c)* is represented lowest in the plane and the most distant *(a)* is represented highest in the plane. Their proximal projections decrease progressively in size with the square of the distance from the eye. The result is the texture gradient illustrated in the picture plane view. Distal square elements project as trapezoidal elements that get progressively smaller from the bottom of the picture plane to the horizon.

As has been noted, Gibson assumed that the ground plane had special importance in the evolution of the visual system because people (and some animals) walked on the ground. Nevertheless, it is important to note that similar changes in the size and shape of optical texture units take place in all surfaces that are viewed at a slant. For example, the optical texture elements in a vertical wall viewed at a slant are compressed in the horizontal dimension (see figure 9.6). In general, surfaces may be slanted at any angle and the compression in the optical texture may be in any dimension corresponding to the angle of slant.

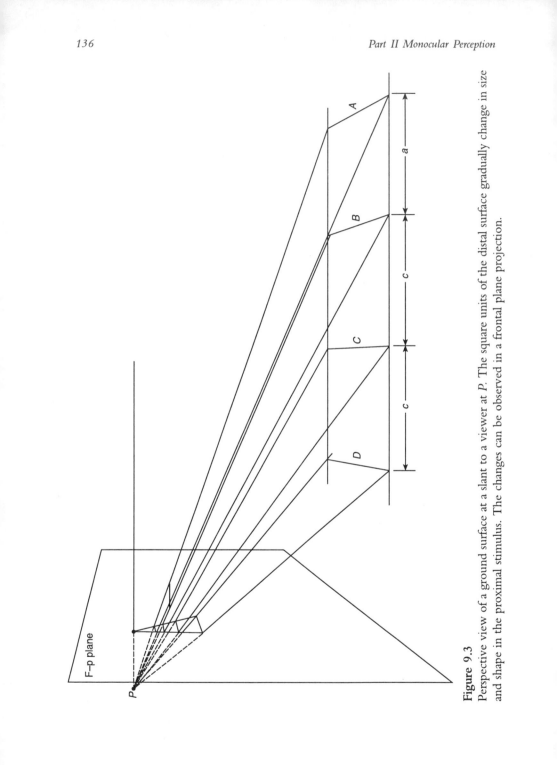

Figure 9.3
Perspective view of a ground surface at a slant to a viewer at *P*. The square units of the distal surface gradually change in size and shape in the proximal stimulus. The changes can be observed in a frontal plane projection.

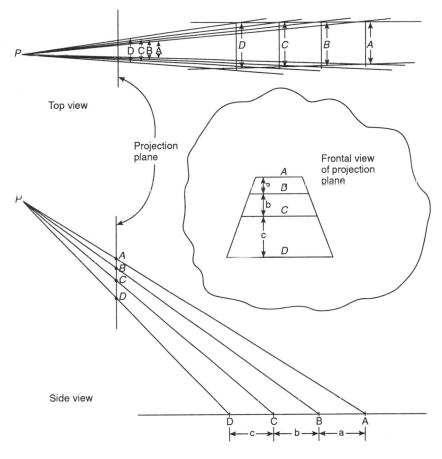

Figure 9.4
Top, side, and picture plane views of the surface in figure 9.3. The lateral dimensions of the square texture elements *(A, B, C, D)* are foreshortened in the proximal stimulus. The depth dimensions of the square texture elements *(a, b, c)* are compressed in the proximal stimulus.

Obviously, *slant perception* is central to Gibson's theory. Optical texture gradients are higher-order variables of stimulation that provide the basis for the perception of surface orientation; i.e., the gradient is the stimulus for the perception of a surface-at-a-slant (Gibson, 1950a, 1950b, 1979; Rosinski & Levine, 1976; Vickers, 1971). Experimental tests generally find that texture gradients produce the perception of a receding surface. However, the measured slant is frequently less than the optically specified slant (see Epstein & Park, 1963; Flock, 1964a, 1964b; Gibson, 1950b; Hochberg, 1971, for reviews). While this evidence might be damaging in evaluating a cue in isolation, in the approach stressing ecological optics, the role of the texture gradient must be evaluated differently. First, experiments using static gradients produced by fixed surfaces are not relevant. In Gibson's view, static stimulation is artificial. Furthermore, in ecological optics, optical texture only provides some of the information in the optic array. Therefore, in Gibson's view, it is not surprising that perception is not completely accurate when the superstimulus is subjected to too fine an analysis.

The Ground and Perceptual Constancy

Distance and the Layout of Space

The natural scene usually consists of objects arranged on a ground. The objects appear at different distances and in different directions from the viewer (egocentric distance and direction), and the distances between objects (exocentric distance) may also vary (Haber, 1986). The texture in a homogeneously textured surface provides a *uniform scale* across the surface. Thus, in a sense, the texture element is a unit of measurement in the surface. Although this holds for any surface, it is most often stressed with respect to the ground where the scale provided by the texture can determine the perceived distance from the observer to a point, the perceived distance between points, and even the perceived size of objects that rest on the surface.

Perceived Size and Distance

Objects that rest on the ground intersect the ground surface and occlude portions of it. The size of the units of texture in the texture gradient produced by the ground are different at different vertical positions in the picture plane. Therefore, the relative change of size and shape of the units in the texture gradient of the ground provides a scale for the space in which the objects are perceived.

These relationships are illustrated in figure 9.5. The ground is represented by a uniform optical texture gradient and a horizon. Three objects occlude a portion of the ground in the picture plane. The visual angle subtended by object *A* is equal to that of object *B* and larger than that of object *C*. Object *B* is higher in the plane than *A* and at the same height as *C*. If the ground were not present, the perceived sizes of *A*, *B*, and *C* would be based purely on visual angle size: $A = B > C$.

With the ground present, the perceived size of the objects is determined relative to the ground: $A = C < B$, and the perceived distance of the objects is $A < B = C$. *A* and *C* appear equal in size in the horizontal dimension because they occlude the same proportion of texture (slightly more than one unit in the figure) and *B* appears larger because it occludes more than three units of texture. *A* and *C* appear to be the same height because the ratio of their sizes is the same as that of the ratio of the texture elements that they occlude. *B* looks higher because its ratio greatly exceeds this. *B* and *C* appear to be at the same distance because their lower contours are at the same relative height in the picture plane. *A* appears closer because it is lower in the the picture plane than *B* and *C*.

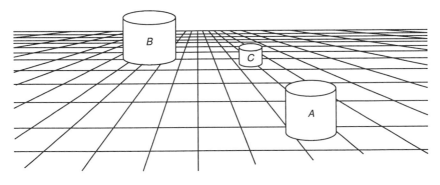

Figure 9.5
Three objects occlude a portion of the ground in the picture plane. The solid visual angle subtended by object *A* is equal to that of object *B* and larger than that of object *C*. The perceived sizes and perceived distances of the objects are determined relative to the texture of the ground: $A = C < B$ for size, and $A < B = C$ for distance.

Size Constancy

Figure 9.6 illustrates the role of the optical texture gradient with respect to three objects *(A, B, C)* in a room with textured floor and walls. The objects in figure 9.6a subtend different visual angles but the difference is proportional to the gradient of texture. These relationships in the proximal stimulus produce perceived size constancy for objects at different perceived distances: $s_A = s_B = s_C$ and $d_A < d_B < d_C$. Thus, size constancy is a consequence of the scale of space.

The objects in figure 9.6b subtend the same visual angles. However, in this case, their angular sizes do not correspond to the changes in the gradient of texture. The objects appear to be at the same distances as those in figure 9.6a because they intersect the texture gradient of the floor (ground) at the same relative heights in the picture plane. However, inverting the relationships between visual angle and the size of the texture unit results in a perception of three different-sized objects: $s_A < s_B < s_C$.

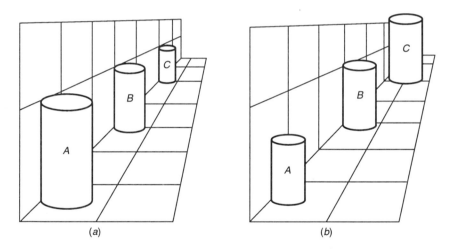

(a)   (b)

Figure 9.6
Three objects *(A, B, C)* in a textured room. (a) The objects subtend different visual angles that are proportional to the gradient of texture. The result is perceived size constancy for objects at different perceived distances: $s_A = s_B = s_C$ and $d_A < d_B < d_C$. (b) Objects *A*, *B*, and *C* subtend the same visual angles. Therefore, they do not correspond to the gradient of texture. The objects appear to be at the same distances as those in (a) because they intersect the texture gradient of the floor at the same relative heights in the picture plane. However, these proximal size relationships result in a perception of objects of different sizes: $s_A < s_B < s_C$.

Intersection of Surfaces

The optic array may contain many areas with different texture gradients. If these areas are perceived as surfaces at slants, they will appear to intersect either at a corner or at an edge. The perceptions of a corner or an edge are produced by different proximal patterns.

Corner

Figure 9.7 shows the proximal pattern that leads to the perception of a corner. The upper portion shows a side view of a distal corner produced by two similar surfaces (i.e., surfaces of the same material) at different slants with respect to a viewer. The lower portion shows the proximal pattern: two areas with the same texture elements but different gradients. This proximal pattern produces the perception of two surfaces meeting at a corner—a surface that has a fold or crease. It does not imply occlusion of any part of the surfaces, only a relative difference in perceived slant. Furthermore, the corner may appear in perception even if it is not present in the proximal pattern, another example of a subjective contour.

Edge

Figure 9.8 shows a proximal pattern that leads to the perception of an edge. The upper portion shows a side view of a distal edge produced by two dissimilar surfaces, one partially occluding the other. To simplify, the surfaces are made of different material and are at the same slant with respect to a viewer. Because there are different elements of texture in the distal surfaces, there are different elements of optical texture in the proximal projections. Because the surfaces are at the same slant with respect to the viewer, the proximal projection has the same gradient of size and shape of the texture elements. The lower portion shows the proximal pattern: two areas with different texture elements but the same gradients. This proximal pattern produces the perception of two parallel surfaces, one occluding a portion of the other. The perception of a relative position difference includes occlusion of the far surface by the near surface. In this case, the edge that appears between the surfaces belongs to the nearer surface and may appear in perception even if it is not present in the proximal pattern, another example of a subjective contour.

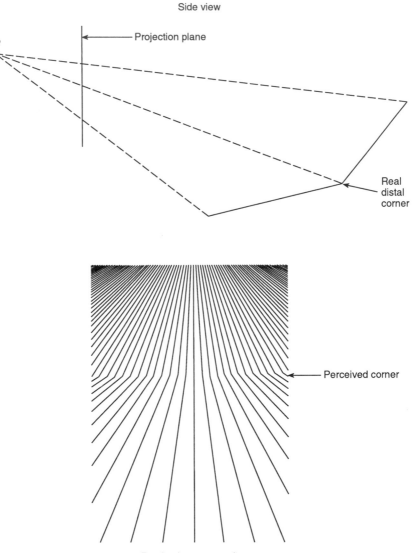

Side view

Projection plane

P

Real distal corner

Perceived corner

Proximal representation

Figure 9.7
Side view of a distal corner produced by two similar surfaces at different slants with respect to a viewer. The proximal pattern is illustrated in the lower portion: two areas with the same texture elements but different gradients.

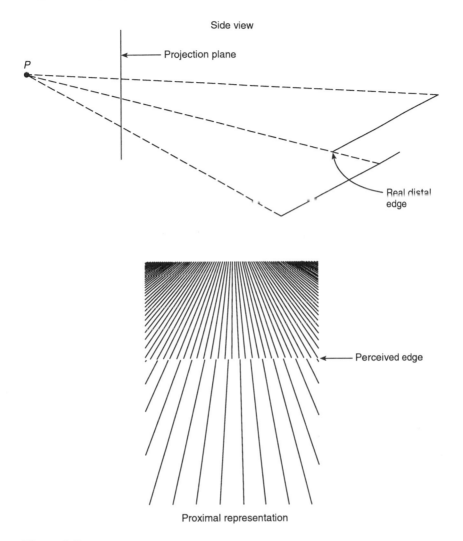

Figure 9.8
Side view of a distal edge produced by two dissimilar surfaces, one partially occluding the other. To simplify, the surfaces are made of different materials and are at the same slant with respect to a viewer. The proximal pattern is illustrated in the lower portion: two areas with different texture elements but the same gradient.

Summary

Gibson's ecological optics presents a new analysis of visual stimulation seeking to identify higher-order invariants in stimulation that correlate with specific aspects of perception. Surfaces consist of substances that provide its texture which, in turn, produces the optical texture in the visual stimulus. When a surface is viewed at a slant, the optical texture contains a gradient, a gradual change in size and shape of texture elements in the optic array. The optical texture gradient is the stimulus for the perception of surface-at-a-slant. The texture gradient from the ground also provides a scale for space. The scale serves as the basis for size-distance perception and underlies perceptual constancy. Differences in texture properties across boundaries provide the basis for the perception of corner and edge.

10

Lateral or Parallactic Motion

The analysis thus far has described situations in which both the viewer and the stimulus are stationary. Of course, this is rarely the case, except in experiments. Natural viewing situations are usually kinetic, involving a moving observer and moving objects. Therefore, the study of motion and movement perception involves analyses of changing information and requires a distinction between physical motions of objects (including the perceiver) and subjective impressions of movement.

Although normal perception involves physical objects that move and a perceiver who moves in 3D space, to simplify the presentation, the analysis uses a stationary viewer and moving stimuli or a moving viewer with stationary stimuli. Three-dimensional physical motions are separated into frontal plane motions (lateral or parallactic motion), motion in depth (radial motion), and rotations. These components of motion are treated in separate chapters. This chapter describes lateral or parallactic motions; chapter 11 describes motion and movement in depth; and chapter 12 discusses the problem of perceiving the 3D rotation of objects.

The study of lateral or parallactic motion perception can be approached from the same varied points of view as those applied to static perception. This chapter begins with the traditional study of local point stimulation. Using the concept of *optic flow*, it progresses to the analysis of global changes in proximal motion patterns—motion perspective, dynamic occlusion, and continuous perspective transformations.

Motion Parallax

Traditionally, the study of lateral motion begins with the analysis of the motions of points. As a viewer moves laterally, object points at different distances project as retinal points that move laterally with different velocities. This relative motion of proximal points resulting from lateral movement of the observer is *motion parallax*. Figure 10.1 illustrates the proximal motion patterns that are produced by two aligned distal points when a viewer moves from position *A* to position *B*. In the lefthand portion of the figure, a far point *(P_F)* is represented by a small rectangle aligned behind a fixated point *(F)* and, in the righthand portion, a near point *(P_N)* is represented by a small triangle aligned in front of the fixated point.

The respective proximal patterns are illustrated in the lower part of the figure. As the viewer moves from position *A* to position *B,* there is a change in the proximal positions of the far and near points with respect to that of the fixated point. The motions of these points can be described by a vector having direction and velocity. For distal points beyond the fixation point, the proximal projection moves in the same direction as the viewer. This is described as *with motion.* For distal points closer than the fixation point, the proximal projection moves in a direction opposite to that of the viewer. This is described as *against motion.* The angular velocities of the two points are (approximately) inversely proportional to their respective distances from the viewer.

Motion parallax provides information about the relative distance between the distal points. The relative direction of motion of a proximal point (*with* or *against* the motion of the viewer) provides information about the relative position of the point with respect to fixation: A proximal point that moves *with* the viewer appears to be behind the fixation point, and a proximal point that moves *against* the viewer appears to be closer than the fixation point. The egocentric distance from the viewer and the relative perceived distance between two points vary directly with the velocity of the moving proximal points—the greater the velocity, the greater the respective perceived distances (see Braunstein & Tittle, 1988; Ono, Rivest, & Ono, 1986; and Regan, 1991, for reviews).

Optic Flow, Velocity Gradients

Gibson (1950a, 1966, 1968, 1979) defined the *optic array* as the pattern of light intensities over the visual field. The optic array changes with physical motions of external objects and with movement of the viewer. *Optic flow* is the spatiotemporal change in the structure of the optic array. Gibson noted that optic flow is different from *retinal flow* because the latter may contain

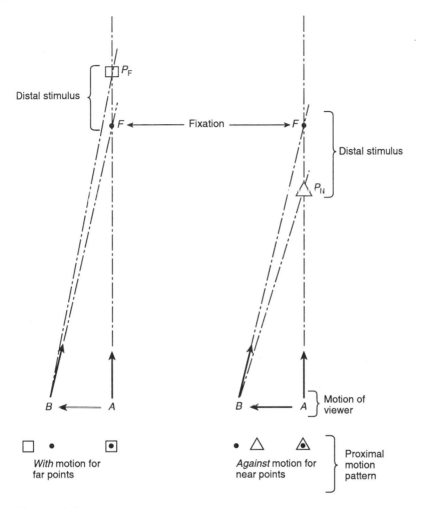

Figure 10.1
Motion parallax patterns produced by two aligned points for a viewer moving
laterally. A point *(P_F)* more distant than the fixation point *(F)* produces *with motion*
in the proximal stimulus, and a point *(P_N)* closer to the viewer than the fixation
point produces *against motion* in the proximal stimulus.

influences from eye movements. Both optic and retinal flow are typically represented as instantaneous 2D velocity fields in which each vector represents the instantaneous optical velocity of an environmental element. In general, distal motion or motion of the observer produces a continuous gradient of proximal velocities over the visual field. Thus, in a sense, the moving observer can control the flow. Analyses of differential derivatives that describe the optic flow field in terms of divergence, curl, and shear components are presented in chapter 12 (Koenderink, 1985, 1986; Koenderink & van Doorn, 1976; Longuet-Higgins & Prazdny, 1980; Regan, 1986b).

In cue theories, the relative velocity between proximal points (motion parallax) is assumed to be a cue to the relative perceived distance between the points. In flow theories, points in the optic array usually appear to be embedded in surfaces. The relative perceived distance from the fixation plane is a function of the relative parallactic velocity in the flow pattern: Slow-moving points appear to be close to the depth of the fixation plane; fast-moving points appear to be far from the fixation plane. These factors determine directly the relative perceived position (or slant) of the surface with respect to the fixation plane and to the viewer. In Gibson's view, depth and motion are perceived directly; in other theories, the relative velocities provide information about the total pattern.

Motion Perspective

In Gibson's (1950a, 1966, 1968, 1979) analysis, observer motion produces displacement in the position of the eye (*station point*) relative to the illuminated environment. The simultaneous changes that occur for all proximal points can be described as *flow patterns*. Figure 10.2 shows these relationships for a viewer moving from right to left looking at point *F*. The arrows represent vectors that describe the directions and velocities of the proximal projections of the distal points. This transformation of the entire array of ambient light resulting from movement of the viewer is *motion perspective* (Gibson, 1950a; Gibson, Olum, & Rosenblatt, 1955).

As in motion parallax, the direction of change of each point in the proximal stimulus is determined by its distal position with respect to the fixation point. All distal points beyond the fixation plane produce *with motion* in the proximal stimulus, and all points closer than the fixation plane produce *against motion* in the proximal stimulus. Points also differ in the velocities of their motion. The greater the distal distance between a point

ʌ

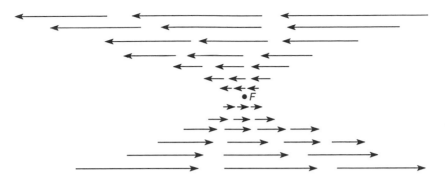

Figure 10.2
Parallactic changes in the scene as a viewer moves laterally are represented as a vector flow field. The direction of the arrows corresponds to the *with* and *against motion* of points farther from or nearer to the viewer than the fixation plane, respectively. The length of the arrows represents their relative proximal velocity.

and the fixation point, the greater the velocity in the proximal flow pattern; the closer a point is to the fixation plane, the smaller the velocity in the proximal flow pattern. Therefore, the total proximal pattern contains motion perspective in the form of a gradient of velocities with zero velocity at the fixation plane. In a sense, motion perspective is a parallactic flow pattern that represents a generalization of motion parallax from two points to the entire optic flow field.

According to Gibson (1950a, 1966, 1979), motion perspective produces the perception of subjective movement, not object motion. This is an experience of moving in a rigid world. Moreover, motion perspective produced by the motion of the viewer produces change in the entire texture pattern of the ambient optic array. In contrast, the motion of objects produces perspective changes in part of the optic array.

Figure 10.3 illustrates the proximal changes when a viewer looks at a scene, in this case, a person in front of a house with a tree behind it. The viewer moves continuously from position *P1* to *P5* while maintaining fixation on the house. The tree is behind the fixation plane, and its projection in the proximal stimulus moves in the same direction as the viewer *(with motion)*. The person is closer to the viewer than the fixation plane and its projection in the proximal stimulus moves in a direction opposite to that of the viewer *(against motion)*. This pattern of change in the positions of the objects in the proximal stimulus produces perceived relative depth differences among the objects. The person appears to be in front of the house and the tree appears to be behind the house.

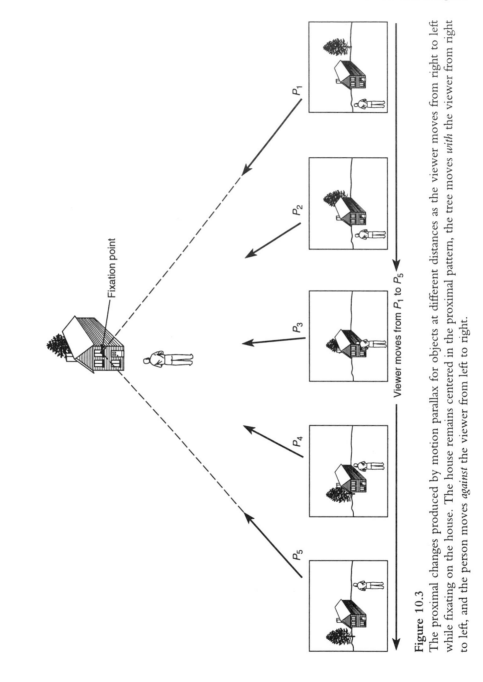

Figure 10.3
The proximal changes produced by motion parallax for objects at different distances as the viewer moves from right to left while fixating on the house. The house remains centered in the proximal pattern, the tree moves *with* the viewer from right to left, and the person moves *against* the viewer from left to right.

Motion parallax has been studied using both fixed and moving observers. In experimental situations with fixed observers, motion parallax produced perceptions of rigid 3D surfaces but they were frequently ambiguous (Braunstein, 1966, 1968; Braunstein & Tittle, 1988; Gibson & Carel, 1952; Gibson, Gibson, Smith, & Flock, 1959). Rogers and Graham (1979) produced unambiguous perceptions from motion parallax by linking it to the motions of the observer and/or the stimulus field. That is, unambiguous depth perception occurred when the motion parallax on a stationary stimulus screen was linked to the sideways motion of an observer's head, or when the parallactic stimulus motion was linked to a moving stimulus field viewed with the head stationary. Rogers and Graham (1979) concluded that ambiguous perceptions were found in earlier studies because stationary displays and stationary observers were used; and these are situations in which no information is available about the relative motion of observer and stimulus field.

Figure 10.4 illustrates how Braunstein and Tittle (1988) incorporated these two components of parallactic information into a single stimulus field. The stimulus consisted of dots moving back and forth in a small window that could move across a large computer screen. To calculate the velocity field within the window, Braunstein and Tittle started with a field of alternate bands moving in opposite directions, a pattern similar to that used by Rogers and Graham (1979). To this pattern, they added a vector representing the velocity of the monitor. The new pattern contained alternate bands moving at different velocities that defined the flow field relative to the observer (head moving left or monitor moving right in the figure).

Thus, the new stimulus carried information about both the relative motion of dot elements in the projected velocity field and the relative motion between the observer's head and the field. The motion parallax flow field constructed in this way produced unambiguous relative depth perception. Braunstein and Tittle (1988) concluded that head motion or monitor motion must be added to motion parallax only if the flow field is ambiguous. When the stimulus field contains information relative to the observer, motion parallax reliably produces the perception of surfaces in ordered depth (Braunstein & Tittle, 1988). Furthermore, motion parallax provides reliable information for detecting the number of surfaces at different distances, their relative depth, and the sign of the depth (Andersen, 1989).

Rogers and Graham (1982, 1985) noted the similarity between stereopsis and motion parallax: *Stereopsis* is based on small differences between

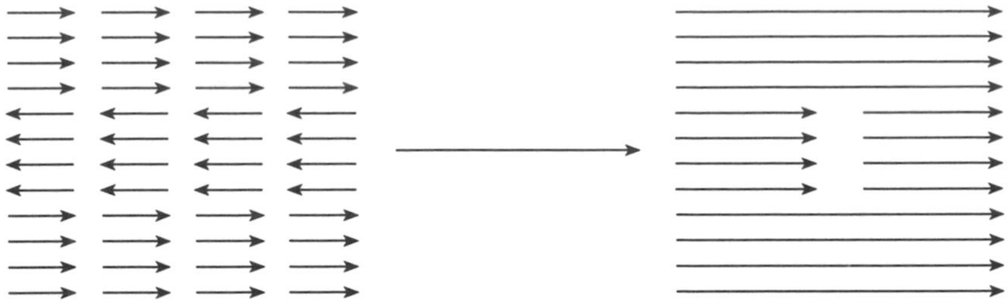

Figure 10.4
A motion parallax field can be combined with a vector representing the velocity of the monitor to produce a flow pattern relative to the viewer (Braunstein & Tittle, 1988). The fields are illustrated for the head moving to the left or the monitor moving to the right.

two simultaneously present half-images, and motion parallax is based on small differences or displacements between two successive monocular images. Furthermore, both approximate an inverse square law (Ono, Rivest, & Ono, 1986). Binocular disparity is given by equation 3.1, a relationship that can be used to calculate motion parallax by substituting values where d = the distance between the points, D = the distance from the observer to the stimulus, and A = the extent of head movement.

In two experiments, Ono, Rivest, and Ono (1986) studied the relationship between motion parallax and absolute distance information, the spatial separation between the observer and the display. Observers reported the apparent depth within the stimulus at two viewing distances (40 and 80 cm) with the extent of motion parallax held constant. The stimulus was similar to that of Rogers and Graham (1979) with side-to-side head motion yoked to the screen. Viewers manually adjusted the distance between two wooden rods to match the apparent depth between peaks and troughs of a perceived corrugated surface. The results showed that viewing distance affected apparent depth even though the extent of parallax was held constant. However, the values only approximated the inverse square law which predicts a 4:1 ratio of apparent depth when the viewing distance is doubled. In the experiment, the mean apparent depth at 80 cm was 2.6 times larger than that at 40 cm.

Ono, Rivest, and Ono (1986) concluded that the visual system calibrates motion parallax information according to absolute distance information (e.g., from accommodation, convergence, vertical angle-of-regard, familiar size, relative distance cues, and other information such as the viewer's translational velocity). They mapped the range of this calibration with measurements at 40, 80, 160, and 320 cm and a wide range of parallax. Observers described their experiences qualitatively as a rigid 3D surface without motion, a corrugated surface rotating along a vertical axis, or a flat rotating surface. Ono, Rivest, and Ono (1986) found that, as distance increased, the perception of a rigid 3D surface was gradually accompanied by the perception of rocking motion, and perception of depth was gradually replaced by perceived motion in some trials at 320 cm. Mean apparent depths were proportional to viewing distance at 40 and 80 cm but not at greater distances. Thus, the depth constancy at the shorter distances fell off rapidly as distance increased.

Dynamic Occlusion

A natural scene contains many surfaces at different distances from the observer. With static viewing, a near surface may occlude a portion of a more distant surface. When the viewer changes position, or when the surfaces move relative to one another, their representations in the optic array undergo changes in the parallactic occlusion patterns. The proximal patterns associated with these events are illustrated in figure 10.5. For a stationary viewer, it represents the proximal events produced when a surface moves across the field of view from right to left. The figure also represents the proximal events for a person moving from left to right fixating beyond a fixed object in front of a ground.

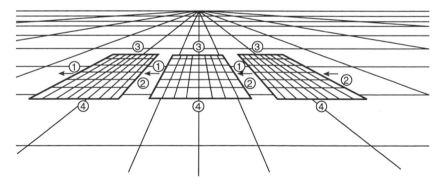

Figure 10.5
Relative motions of surfaces: Optical texture from the more distant surface (the ground) is progressively covered (deleted) and uncovered (accreted) along the boundaries of the near object that are not parallel to the motion (edges 1 and 2, respectively). The edges parallel to the motion (edges 3 and 4) cut or shear the texture.

The proximal pattern changes simultaneously in three ways in this configuration (Gibson, 1950a, 1966, 1979). First, the texture of the more distant object is progressively covered *(deleted)* and uncovered *(accreted)* along the boundaries of the near object that are not parallel to the motion. Thus, the texture of the ground continuously disappears at the leading edge of the near surface and progressively appears at the trailing edge of the near surface. At the edges parallel to the motion, the sides of the near object cut the occluded texture. Second, the texture of the object moves at a proximal speed different from that of the ground. Third, the moving texture points form blur lines that have different lengths within the object and the surround (Regan, 1986a).

Dynamic occlusion may not be necessary for the perception of relative depth from motion parallax. When relative motion and dynamic occlusion were made to supply opposite relative depth information between two planes, relative motion determined perceived relative depth for small depth separations, and dynamic occlusion determined relative perceived depth for large separations (Ono, Rogers, Ohmi, & Ono, 1988).

Continuous Perspective Transformations

A stationary surface at a slant to a viewer projects onto the proximal stimulus as a perspective transformation of the outline shape of the surface. When the viewer moves around the stationary surface, or when the distal surface is in motion, there is a continuous change of the perspective transformation in the proximal stimulus. Figure 10.6 illustrates the perspective transformations produced when a person moves around a stationary table. The rectangular tabletop projects as a trapezoid in the proximal stimulus. As the viewer moves, the shape of the projected trapezoid changes continuously.

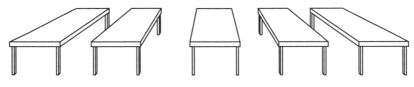

Figure 10.6
Perspective transformations produced when a viewer moves around a stationary table. The rectangular tabletop projects to the proximal stimulus as a trapezoid that changes in shape continuously.

Perspective transformations are discussed in more detail in chapter 11 in the context of perceiving rotating objects.

Summary

This chapter described the stimulus produced when a viewer moves laterally or when stimuli move in the frontal plane. Motion parallax, the relative motion of proximal points produced by such movements, results in the perception of relative depth between the points. Motion perspective is the parallactic change over the entire optic array. This optic flow pattern produces the perception of relative depth among the various parts of the visual field. When the viewer of the scene moves, dynamic occlusion occurs—there is progressive deletion and accretion along the edges of the nearer object. Finally, perspective transformations occur in the shapes of surfaces.

11

Motion in Depth

The motion of an object that is moving directly toward or away from a viewer is loosely described as *radial motion* (Ames, 1955; Ittelson, 1951a). Obviously, all points on an object cannot simultaneously follow a path along a radius to the observer's egocenter. Radial motion simply separates the egocentric motions of objects from other types of motions.

The Stimulus

Although radially moving objects are represented by expanding or contracting proximal areas, to simplify the discussion, the analysis begins with radial motion of a distal line.

Size-Change

The stimulus relationships for a single line (a contour or edge) moving radially are illustrated in the upper portion of figure 11.1. A distal line of fixed size *(S)* moves directly toward a viewer *(D₁ to D₂)* over time interval t_1 to t_2, producing a proximal line *(retinal extent)* increasing in size. This proximal stimulus can be described as an increasing visual angle α_1 to α_2. The lower portion of the figure shows a frontal view of the projection plane illustrating this change in visual angle size. A distal line moving directly away from the viewer produces a decreasing proximal size.

The one-dimensional change in the proximal stimulus is an increasing or decreasing *size-change* stimulus. The changing size of a linear retinal extent can also be represented by the motion of dots at the endpoints of an invisible line. Thus, the changing separation between two points can also be described as a size-change stimulus (for example, see Börjesson and von Hofsten's [1972, 1973] analysis of dot-motions in chapter 12).

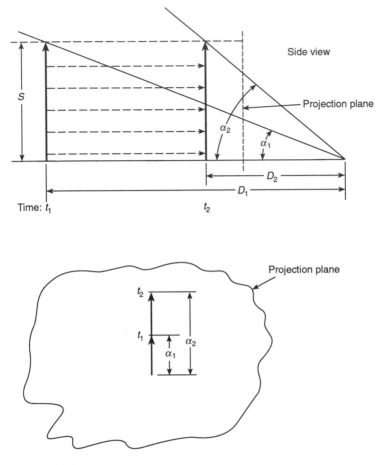

Figure 11.1
A size-change stimulus. A distal line of fixed size *(S)* moves directly toward a viewer
(D₁ to D₂) over time interval *t₁* to *t₂*, producing an increase in proximal size (visual
angle: α₁ to α₂).

An increasing or decreasing size-change pattern is an ambiguous stimulus when presented alone. That is, it does not produce a unique perceptual
outcome. It may be seen as a contour in the frontal plane that is increasing
or decreasing in size, as a rigid contour *(rod)* moving radially in depth or
rotating in depth about a point, or as a rigid contour folding into a V–shape
consisting of two rigid components (Börjesson & von Hofsten, 1972; Hershenson, 1993b; Johansson & Jansson, 1968).

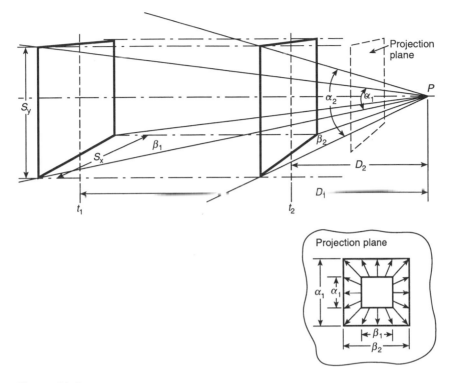

Figure 11.2
An expansion stimulus. A distal surface of fixed size $(S_x \times S_y)$ moves directly toward the viewer (radially: D_1 to D_2) over time interval t_1 to t_2, producing a symmetrical increase in proximal stimulus area.

Expansion/Contraction (E/C)

The proximal changes associated with radial motion of a surface are illustrated in figure 11.2. When a distal surface of fixed size $(S_x \times S_y)$ moves directly toward the viewer (radially: D_1 to D_2) over time interval t_1 to t_2, it produces a symmetrically increasing proximal area; when it moves directly away from the viewer, it produces a symmetrically decreasing proximal area. The lower portion of the figure illustrates an *expansion pattern*—a frontal plane projection that increases in solid visual angle $(\alpha_1 \times \beta_1$ to $\alpha_2 \times \beta_2)$. A decrease in solid visual angle is a *contraction pattern*. If the motion is not directly toward or away from the viewer, the expansion or contraction pattern is asymmetrical.

Figure 11.3 shows the visual angle subtended by an object of fixed size as a function of distance from the viewer. Visual angle varies inversely with

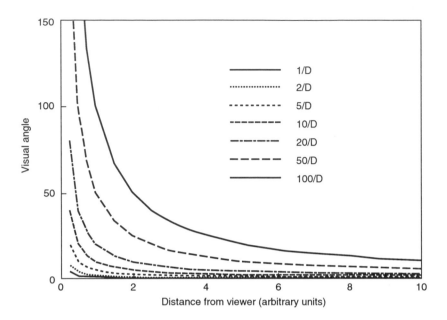

Figure 11.3
Visual angle subtended by an object of fixed size varies inversely as a function of distance from the viewer. For an object approaching at a uniform velocity, the increase is gradual at first and becomes quite rapid as it nears the viewer.

distance, i.e., it increases as the object approaches and decreases as the object recedes. For an object approaching at a uniform velocity, the increase is gradual at first and becomes quite rapid as it nears the viewer. Furthermore, the proximal subtense changes at different rates for different points on the surface. Points on the surface that are close to the line of sight of the viewer increase their proximal separation more slowly than those that are more distant from the line of sight. In other words, for an approaching surface, there is a gradient in the increase of proximal distances that increases from the line of sight outward. In general, the rapid increase in visual angle size for an approaching near object is described as *looming*. Although the geometrical relationships are reversed for a receding object, there is no single descriptive term for the corresponding stimulus.

The proximal gradient is represented in the expansion of the flow pattern in the optic array. The texture of a surface projects as optical velocity vectors that radiate outward (inward) from a focus of expansion (contraction) in the optical flow pattern. Figure 11.4 shows an optical expansion pattern generated by a viewer walking forward or an object moving toward

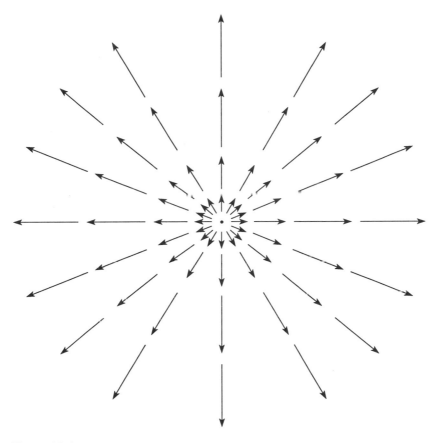

Figure 11.4
An optical expansion pattern generated by an approaching object or by a viewer
walking forward. The vectors in the optical flow pattern radiate from a focal point
and increase in size (velocity) the farther they are from this point.

the viewer. The optical flow pattern consists of vectors radiating from a
focal point and increasing in velocity (size) the farther they are from this
point. There is also a relationship between the E/C pattern and the background texture. As an object approaches a viewer, it occludes more and
more of the background. This relationship is represented in the proximal
stimulus as an expansion pattern with progressive *deletion* of background
texture at the edges of the object. When an object moves directly away
from a viewer, background texture is progressively uncovered. This relationship is represented in the proximal stimulus as a contracting pattern with
the *accretion* of background texture at the edges of the object.

Apparent Object Motions

A proximal expansion pattern produces the perception of a rigid object moving directly toward the viewer, and a proximal contraction pattern produces the perception of a rigid object moving directly away from the viewer (Ames, 1955; Gibson, 1950a; Ittelson, 1951a; Schiff, 1965). A looming stimulus produces eye-blink, head-turn, or retreat responses in a wide variety of species, including human neonates, and lower organisms such as octopus, chickens, and fish (Börjesson & von Hofsten, 1973; Braunstein, 1976; Gibson, 1950a; Hershenson, 1982, 1993b; Johansson, 1977; Koenderink, 1986; Schiff, 1965; Swanston & Gogel, 1986). On the basis of these responses, it is likely that the various organisms perceive a rigid object moving toward them as being on a direct collision course. That is, they demonstrate size and shape constancy.

Kinetic Invariance Hypothesis
The rule governing the relationship between perceived size and perceived distance for a static stimulus is the *static SDIH* (see chapter 8). The SDIH asserts that, for a given visual angle, the perception will be one of the family of equivalent configurations that could have produced the proximal stimulus. The perceptions associated with a changing proximal stimulus, an expansion/contraction pattern, suggest that a different invariance formulation is necessary. This is the kinetic size–distance invariance hypothesis, or simply the *kinetic invariance hypothesis* (KIH). It asserts that a proximal expansion or contraction pattern, i.e., an increasing or decreasing solid visual angle, produces the perception of an object of constant size (a rigid object) changing its perceived radial distance.

The proximal-perceptual relations implied by the KIH are illustrated in figure 11.5 (to simplify, the discussion is limited to one meridian of change). Given a proximal expansion pattern $(\alpha_1$ to $\alpha_2)$, a rigid object of perceived size s (where $s = K$) appears to move toward the viewer over a perceived distance, d_1 to d_2. Given a proximal contraction pattern, a rigid object of perceived size s appears to move away from the viewer over a perceived distance, d_2 to d_1. Thus, in the kinetic case, perceived size remains constant while perceived distance varies. The experimental evidence shows that this outcome is almost invariably the case (Ames, 1955; Börjesson & von Hofsten, 1973; Braunstein, 1976; Gibson, 1950a, 1966, 1979; Hershenson, 1982, 1993b; Ittelson, 1951a; Johansson, 1977; Koenderink, 1986;

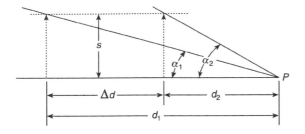

Figure 11.5
Proximal-perceptual relationships underlying the kinetic invariance hypothesis:
Given a proximal expansion pattern $(\alpha_1$ to $\alpha_2)$, a rigid object appears to move
toward the viewer from d_1 to d_2; given a proximal contraction pattern $(\alpha_2$ to $\alpha_1)$, a
rigid object appears to move away from the viewer from d_2 to d_1.

Schiff, 1965; Swanston & Gogel, 1986). Thus, the KIH is different from
the static case where perceived size and perceived distance vary simultaneously. Nevertheless, instantaneous time samples of perceptions in the kinetic
situation do satisfy the SDIH.

KIH and Size Constancy
The analysis of perceived size for radially moving objects reveals at least two
components to size constancy: perceived linear size and perceived rigidity
(Hershenson, 1992a). *Perceived linear size* is the quantitative experience that
an object has a specific metric size, whereas *perceived rigidity* is the qualitative
experience that an object has not changed in size (has not grown larger or
smaller) over time.

   The difference between perceived rigidity and perceived linear size is
illustrated in figure 11.6. It shows that the same change in retinal extent
(visual angle) can produce two different perceptions with regard to the
metric size of the object, but still yield perceived rigidity. In the figure, the
proximal stimulus is represented by a visual angle change $(\Delta\alpha = \alpha_1$ to $\alpha_2)$.
Under the KIH, a given proximal change in solid visual angle appears to be
a rigid object moving in depth.

   Two possible perceived rigid objects are pictured, one of metric size
s_1 and one of metric size s_2. According to the KIH, the proximal stimulus
could be perceived as a rigid object of size s_1 moving toward the viewer
from d_1 to d_2. But the identical proximal stimulus change could be perceived
as a rigid object of metric size s_2 moving from d_3 to d_4. In both cases, the
object appears to be rigid, to move toward the viewer, and to satisfy the
KIH. However, neither the KIH nor the SDIH determines perceived metric

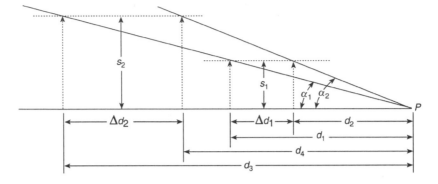

Figure 11.6
The difference between perceived rigidity and perceived metric size. The proximal stimulus is a visual angle change $(\Delta\alpha = \alpha_1$ to $\alpha_2)$. Two possible perceived rigid objects are pictured, one of metric size s_1 and one of metric size s_2. The perception could be a rigid object of metric size s_1 moving toward the viewer from d_1 to d_2 or a rigid object of metric size s_2 moving from d_3 to d_4. In both cases, the object appears to be rigid, to move toward the viewer, and to satisfy the KIH.

size—it is determined only when additional information is available to the perceptual system. Thus, an object may be perceived as rigid or even as the same metric size at two different distances, but the perception may not be veridical—the perceived size and the distal size may still differ.

Rigidity and the Implicit Scales of Space
The problem presented by the static invariance hypothesis is simply to determine a unique perceived size-distance ratio. The kinetic invariance hypothesis presents a different problem—although rigidity and motion in depth are important features of the perception, neither is contained in the proximal stimulus (Todd, 1982, 1984). The problem is to describe a mechanism that could produce these perceptual qualities.

In one interpretation, the experience of rigidity is attributed to an automatic perceptual mechanism, one whose operation is an essential feature of perceptual system activity. This activity has been described as a *rigidity assumption* (Johansson, 1958, 1977; Ullman, 1979a, 1979b) or a *rigidity constraint* (Hershenson, 1982, 1992a, 1992b). A *rigidity assumption* refers to automatic activity of the visual system that results in the perception of an object whose size is unchanging. Formally, the *rigidity constraint* may be understood as a mechanism that scales perceptual space so as to maintain a constant perceived size. This constancy scaling determines the *implicit scale of space*. A major consequence of this scaling is that, in conjunction with the relationship described by the KIH, the rigidity constraint produces perceived motion in depth. Thus, perceived rigidity and perceived motion in depth are linked by the scaling function and the KIH (Hershenson, 1992a).

Gibson's (1950a, 1966, 1979) interpretation yields three sources of information that are scaled for distance: linear perspective, motion perspective, and binocular disparity. Each source is represented as a gradient that is directly related to the distance of texture elements of distal surfaces. *Linear perspective* and the associated texture gradient of the ground specify a rate of change of size (and shape) with respect to distance, with the viewer's feet as the reference point. *Motion perspective* specifies rates of displacement across the scene, with the point of fixation as the reference. The *gradient of retinal disparity* specifies relative depth, with the point of zero disparity (the fixation point or point of binocular convergence) as the reference (Haber, 1978, 1983; Haber & Hershenson, 1980).

The three scales specify the spatial arrangement of the scene simultaneously over the entire visual field. That is, each has scalar properties that describe rules relating position in the proximal stimulus to position in the perceived 3D world extending away from the viewer. This is a unique property of the scales that makes them different from the properties of the local pictorial depth cues. Therefore, as the viewer moves about, the scales of space provide correlated information about the relative positions in space of objects and ground. This information may be used as the basis for metric size and shape constancy as well as for position and direction constancy (Haber, 1983; Hershenson, 1992a).

Movement of Perceiver

Visual sensitivity to the expansion and contraction of texture has been studied as it relates to the perception of observer motion. For example, sensitivity to the differential rate of expansion of texture permits accurate sensing of small differences among distances of textured depth planes for a person moving forward (Beverley & Regan, 1983; Regan & Beverley, 1982, 1983).

Heading and Focus of Expansion

The center of expansion of the optic array may be used to guide locomotion. When an observer moves forward and fixates the impact point, that point remains stationary in the optic flow pattern. This point is the *focus of expansion* or *focus of flow* of the optic array. As illustrated in figure 11.4, other distal points are represented by proximal points that move radially, i.e., away from the focus of expansion with greater rates of motion the farther the distance from the impact point. This pattern also occurs if the gaze is maintained at a fixed angle to a distant point.

Gibson (1950a, 1959; Gibson & Gibson, 1957) assumed that information for visual self-guidance is available in the optic flow pattern. He suggested that the focus of flow may supply the information used to guide locomotion when it corresponds to the viewer's destination. Indeed, when a viewer is moving in a stationary world, the focus of expansion lies in the direction of movement if the viewer is looking in that direction (Regan & Beverley, 1979, 1982). However, the proximal flow pattern of a moving observer frequently does not contain a focus of expansion that coincides with the destination (Regan & Beverley, 1982). The patterns differ, for example, when the observer moves forward but does not look at the destination, or looks at some other point in the field. When this happens, the eyes rotate continuously as the viewer moves and this motion adds a translational velocity component to the entire proximal velocity field. That is, the radial expansion pattern produced by the motion forward has an additional translational component due to the change in fixation.

Thus, the change in the flow pattern may change the focus of expansion so that it no longer coincides with the destination of the movement (Koenderink, 1985; Koenderink & van Doorn, 1976; Regan & Beverley, 1982; Richards, 1975). Nevertheless, the perception of heading over a ground plane is accurate—humans can distinguish the direction of heading from the direction of some other environmental reference point to an accuracy of 1 deg of visual angle (Warren, Morris, & Kalish, 1988), suggesting that the flow field is decomposed into translatory and rotary components (Van den Berg, 1992).

Time-to-Contact and Time-to-Passage

When an object moves directly toward a viewer or the viewer moves directly toward the object, or both, the viewer and the object are on a collision course. The *time-to-contact (TTC)* is defined as the instantaneous distance to the object divided by the speed of approach (Lee, 1976, 1980). Following the lead of Gibson (1950a, 1966), a number of studies found evidence that judged TTC is correlated with *tau (τ)*, the reciprocal of the relative rate of dilation of the visual angle (see Bootsma & Oudejans, 1993;

Kaiser & Mowafy, 1993; and Tresilian, 1991, for reviews). If α is the visual angle between two points on a surface patch that is moving toward the observer with a constant velocity, the *TTC* is specified by the reciprocal of the instantaneous rate of dilation of α, $(d\alpha/dt)/\alpha$, and the reciprocal is *tau* (Lee, 1976):

$$\tau = \alpha/(d\alpha/dt). \tag{11.1}$$

If the instantaneous solid visual angle Ω subtended by the entire patch is considered (Lee & Young, 1985), then:

$$\tau = 2\Omega/(d\Omega/dt). \tag{11.2}$$

These are examples of *local tau* because they are defined locally without using the global velocity field (Tresilian, 1991). *Global tau* is the optical variable that is more useful in specifying *time-to-passage (TTP)* for off-axis approaches. It is based on features of the velocity field as a whole and requires detection of the focus of expansion (radial outflow) during the observer's forward motion. If θ is the angular extent between an object point and the observer's track vector, *global tau* is given by:

$$\tau_G = \theta/(d\theta/dt). \tag{11.3}$$

Kaiser and Mowafy (1993) reported accurate and robust judgments of *TTP* using *global tau*.

Information for Controlling Activity

Gibson (1950a) described two types of information necessary for controlling activity: *exteroceptive* and *proprioceptive information*. *Exteroception* provides information about the layout of the environment and external objects and events. *Proprioception* is information from receptors in muscles and joints about the acts being performed.

Lee (1974) carried the analysis further by distinguishing between two sources of proprioceptive information: proprioception and exproprioception. In Lee's refined definition, *proprioception* is information about positions and movements of the parts of the body relative to the body, and *exproprioception* is information about the position, orientation, or movement of the body as a whole, or part of the body relative to the environment. Exteroceptive information is used in planning an act relative to the environment; proprioceptive information is used in controlling the act; and exproprioceptive information is used in both planning and control of an act. Stimulation can also be categorized according to the source of change in the proximal pattern. *Exafferent stimulation* describes change in the visual field caused by motion of an object in the environment. *Reafferent stimulation* describes change in the proximal stimulus pattern caused by movements of the viewer (von Holst, 1954).

Visual Kinesthesis

Lishman and Lee (1973) studied the relationships involved in exproprioception in a swinging room. Figure 11.7 shows the experimental situation: a three-walled "room" that could swing back and forth around a small trolley. The walls of the room were patterned. A subject stood erect on the trolley, which could remain stationary or move. The swinging motion of the room produced the same changing visual stimulus (optical flow pattern) as that produced when the subject moved and the room was stationary.

Active and passive conditions were compared. In the passive condition, the subject remained stationary while the room swung. In the active condition, the subject walked toward, or away from, the front wall. For both approach and recession, subjects reported that they were moving in a stationary room. The experience was so compelling that viewers felt as if they were moving even when they were stationary. Lishman and Lee described these results as a strong dominance of visual over mechanical kinesthetic information. Furthermore, the direction of looking was not important, and knowledge of the situation had little effect. Lishman and Lee suggested that the swinging room experiments demonstrate the operation of *exproprioceptive information:* information about the position, orientation, or movement of the body as a whole relative to the environment.

Balance and Stance

Lee and Lishman (1975) proposed three possible sources of proprioceptive information: vestibular, articular, and visual information. They ruled out vestibular input because the effective sensitivity is too low. *Articular information* is the proprioceptive information that results from changes in angles and pressures registered by mechanoreceptors in muscles, joints, and feet, usually associated with movement on firm ground. Visual information is relevant because any movement of the body gives rise to movement in the optic flow field. Presumably these changes in the optic flow field carry information about movement of the body relative to environment.

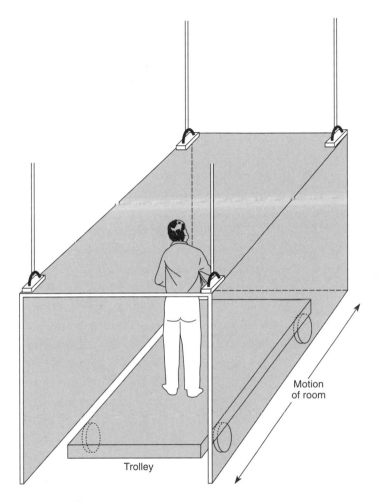

Figure 11.7
Swinging room used by Lishman and Lee (1973; Lee & Lishman, 1975). The walls of the room were patterned. The trolley and room could move forward and backward independently. A subject standing on the trolley could remain stationary or could walk forward and backward.

To investigate these possible inputs, Lee and Lishman attached a "sway meter" to the backs of subjects in the swinging room. In one experiment, four "normal stances" were tested: standing normally on a hard floor, standing on a ramp, standing on a compliant (foam) surface, and standing on one's toes. There were four conditions: eyes open and closed, and front wall of the swinging room near and far. Results showed that the presence of visual information improved the subjects' balance in all cases, i.e., body sway was less with eyes open. Indeed, the subjects' sway followed the changes in the visual information—irregular movements of the room caused visual driving of sway that could not be ignored. The subjects were described as *visual puppets*. Lee and Lishman concluded that visual proprioceptive information was used in controlling balance in all stances.

In a second experiment, the three "impossible stances" illustrated in figure 11.8 were tested. These stances were called impossible because balance was very difficult in these positions. In the first stance *(a)*, the subject stood erect on a 2-by-4 beam. In the "Chaplin" stance *(b)*, the subject stood with feet together and toes pointed outward. In the "pinstripe" stance *(c)*, the subject stood with one leg bent at the knee and crossed over the other leg while holding a briefcase in the extended arm on that side. Subjects were

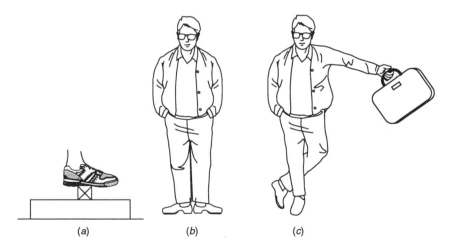

(a)   *(b)*   *(c)*

Figure 11.8
Three stances used by Lee and Lishman (1975) in assessing the visual proprioceptive control of stance. The positions illustrated include (a) standing on a beam; (b) Chaplin stance: heels together, feet pointing in opposite directions; and (c) pinstripe stance: balancing on one leg, other leg bent with foot behind calf, while holding a weight with an extended arm.

not able to balance in any of these positions with their eyes closed, but all balanced for 30 sec with their eyes open. Movement of the swinging room caused all subjects to sway and/or fall.

Lee and Aronson (1974) studied stance and balance in infants who had just started to walk. The infants were placed standing on the floor in the swinging room. When the room moved, the infants swayed and fell in the same direction. Therefore, Lee and Aronson concluded that their balance was visually guided, i.e., they used visual information about body movement to maintain their balance.

Summary

In radial motion, an object moves in depth directly toward or away from a viewer. The proximal stimulus produced by a contour moving radially is an increasing or decreasing size–change pattern. The proximal stimulus produced by a surface moving radially is an expansion or contraction of a proximal area (or of the optic flow) described by a changing solid visual angle. A size-change stimulus does not produce a unique perceptual outcome; an expansion/contraction stimulus invariably produces the perception of a surface moving in depth. The KIH states that an E/C pattern is perceived as a rigid surface changing its perceived radial distance. It suggests that there are implicit scales of space that enter into the processing of perceived size and distance.

Forward and backward movements of the perceiver also produce E/C patterns. The focus of flow of the optic array may be used to determine the direction of motion (heading) of the viewer. Vision also provides exproprioceptive information about the position, orientation, or movement of the body as a whole with respect to the environment. This information is involved in the control of balance and stance.

12

Perceived Object Motions

This chapter describes different approaches to the perception of object motions in space. It begins with the rotating trapezoidal window and the kinetic depth effect, demonstrations that raise fundamental questions about the perception of object motions. The following section describes Johansson's vector analyses, an alternative to the empiricist and psychophysical approaches previously described. The chapter ends with an indication of some modern theoretical directions.

Rotating Stimuli

Rotating objects provide stimuli whose proximal projections change solely as a consequence of the motion of the object. Although different parts of the object may change their locations with respect to the viewer, the axis of rotation does not. Ames's (1951) description of the rotating trapezoidal window clearly defined the problems to be explained.

Rotating Trapezoidal Window

A real rectangular window viewed at a slant has one vertical side closer to the viewer than the other. The window projects onto the frontal plane as a trapezoid (see figure 7.2). Ames (1951, 1955) made this projected window into a real trapezoidal window of wood or metal. It was mounted on a motor and rotated slowly around a vertical axis. When viewed monocularly from about 10 feet, it appeared to be a rectangular window oscillating back and forth through an angle of about 100 deg. As the window approached a position normal to the line of sight, its motion appeared to slow gradually, come to a complete stop, and reverse direction. When viewed from an angle off the midline, the window did not appear rectangular—it was shaped like a trapezium, with the amount of distortion determined by the viewing position.

More complex perceptions were produced by adding objects to the stimulus configuration. One object was a small solid cube attached with a thin rigid rod so that it projected above the short side of the trapezoid. As the trapezoid rotated and appeared to oscillate, the cube appeared to continue its rotational path, leaving the point of attachment and continuing around the window as if it were floating through air. A metal bar was also added, hung through the center of the window. At first, the bar appeared to rotate with the window as it moved. At the critical point when the window began to oscillate (i.e., reversed its direction of motion), the bar and the window appeared almost to collide; the bar appeared to bend around the window, then straighten out, and cut through the window (Ames, 1951, 1955).

The rotating trapezoidal window raises many questions about the perception of objects moving in space. Why does the trapezoidal window appear rectangular? Why does the rotating object appear to oscillate? Why does the window, moving at a constant rate, appear to move at different rates? Ames (1951, 1955) answered these questions by suggesting that perception involves prognostic directives for action involving contributions from the changing stimulus patterns and weighted assumptions from past experience about the possible nature of the objects producing the stimulus. This "transactional" approach is similar to modern empiricist (neo-Helmholtzian) theory in its reliance on experience (Rock, 1977, 1983; Rock & Smith, 1981). It also bears a resemblance to Gibson's (1979) ecological optics in its view of perception as tied to action of the viewer.

Kinetic Depth Effect

Similar questions are raised by the demonstration of the *kinetic depth effect (KDE),* the perception of rigid object motion from a changing (i.e., kinetic) 2D proximal pattern. To study this effect, Wallach and O'Connell (1953) produced a 2D shadow of an object on a screen using the arrangement illustrated in figure 12.1. The screen was essentially a picture plane and the shadow was a 2D perspective representation of the object. The shadow was viewed from the opposite side of the screen so that viewers were unaware of the nature of the object producing the shadow. When the shadow of a wire cube was observed with the stimulus stationary, viewers reported seeing a 2D pattern produced by a flat object. When the wire cube rotated,

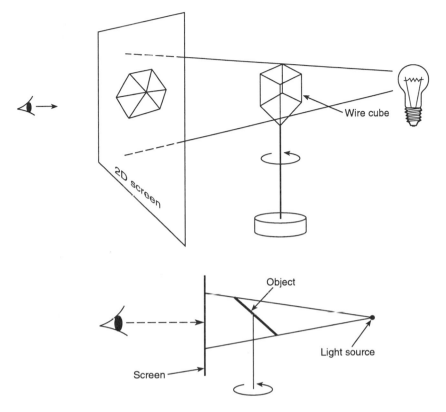

Figure 12.1
Arrangement used by Wallach and O'Connell (1953) to demonstrate the kinetic depth effect. The wire cube, attached to a motor by a rod, can be made to rotate. The shadow of the cube is cast on a screen viewed from the other side.

it produced a moving 2D shadow pattern, a continuous perspective transformation of the cube. Viewers described this changing pattern as a rigid wire cube rotating in depth.

Although Wallach and O'Connell (1953) performed many experiments on the *KDE,* their findings can be summarized by the experiment using a wire **T**. Figure 12.2 illustrates the two proximal patterns compared in this experiment. The upper portion of the figure shows a wire **T** mounted on a vertical rod. In the **T** configuration, the crossbar was perpendicular to the vertical member. When rotated, the proximal pattern it produced was a linear change in the proximal size of the crossbar. This change in a single proximal meridian can be described as a *changing visual angle* or as increasing or decreasing *size-change.* As noted in chapter 11, a size-change stimulus is

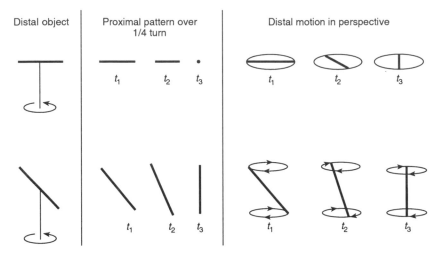

Figure 12.2
The two motion patterns compared in the wire **T** experiment. One stimulus rod is perpendicular to the support and the other is tilted (see text for details).

ambiguous, i.e., there are a number of different perceptions associated with this pattern. It can appear to be a horizontal line changing in size in a frontal plane, a rigid line rotating in depth, a rigid line oscillating in depth, a rigid "V" opening and closing, or a combination of these.

The lower portion of the figure shows the stimulus produced when the crossbar was tilted, i.e., the angle between the vertical member and the bar was no longer 90 deg. When this bar rotated, the shadow it cast was a line that was continuously changing its length and angular position. The figure shows the distal motion of the crossbar in perspective and the proximal pattern over a quarter turn $(t_1$ to $t_3)$. This proximal pattern resulted in the perception of a rigid bar rotating in depth.

Wallach and O'Connell (1953) concluded that the *KDE* depends on simultaneous proximal change in the length and orientation of contours. However, it is not necessary to have a moving contour in the proximal stimulus. A similar effect can be produced with apparent motion of dots (Hershenson, 1992b, 1993b). If the line is replaced with dots at the endpoints, and apparent motion is produced between the beginning and end positions of the continuous motion patterns in figure 12.2, the same differences are observed in the perceptual reports. Therefore, proximal motion per se is not essential for the perception of rigid object motion. What appears to be essential is proximal position change of two or more points (Hershenson, 1992b, 1993b).

The *KDE* can also be explained within other theoretical frameworks. For example, in Gibson's (1950a, 1979) theory of direct perception, simultaneous change in length and orientation defines a continuous perspective transformation, the stimulus for perceived rigid motion in depth. In the context of cognitive theory, Rock and Smith (1981) suggested that the impression of depth results from a process such as inference or problem solving that is not necessarily based on prior experience. They suggested that a transforming proximal stimulus poses the problem of determining what distal event might be producing it. To solve the problem, hypotheses are generated that could fit the stimulus. In the *KDE*, two hypotheses might be considered: a literal solution that mimics the proximal pattern and a "constructive" solution of a rigid object rotating in depth. In this view, perception results from acceptance of one hypothesis over the other.

Stereokinetic Effect

The trapezoidal window and the *KDE* refer to perceived rotations of objects around an axis of rotation in the frontal plane. If the axis of rotation is the line of sight, rigid 3D objects are usually not perceived. One exception to this, the *stereokinetic effect (SKE),* is illustrated in figure 12.3. A stimulus consisting of off-center closed concentric contours is rotated around the center of the disc (outer circle). Viewers report a vivid impression of depth—a cone appears to oscillate about a vertical axis (Caudek & Proffitt, 1993; Musatti, 1924; Proffitt, Rock, Hecht, & Schubert, 1992; Wallach, Weisz, & Adams, 1956; Zanforlin, 1988). Similar explanations have generally been proposed for the *KDE* and *SKE* (Caudek & Proffitt, 1993; Proffitt, Rock, Hecht, & Schubert, 1992).

Johansson's Vector Analysis

Johansson (1950, 1964, 1970, 1973, 1974a, 1974b, 1978a, 1978b) proposed that elements in motion in the proximal stimulus are treated as related to each other in perception, i.e., motion stimulation is relational. He described proximal motions using vectors representing the direction and magnitude of the motion of proximal points. Johansson suggested that the visual system performed an analysis of the proximal motion vectors resulting in a

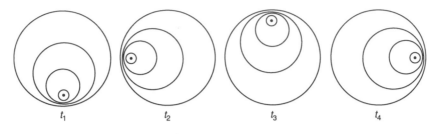

Figure 12.3
The stereokinetic effect. A disc containing embedded nonconcentric circles rotates around its center. Viewers report seeing an asymmetrical 3D cone rotating around the center point.

relationship between the proximal stimulus and perception that he described as an inverse projective geometry. This analysis is achieved by the application of automatic rules for organizing perceptions: unity, rigidity, and the minimum principle.

The *unity principle* asserts that equal components of simultaneous proximal motion vectors in the same direction are perceived as motion of a *unit*. The *rigidity principle* asserts that equal motions in a series of simultaneous proximal elements automatically connect these elements as *rigid* perceptual units. Equal vectors in different orientations yield perceived motion in depth. Thus, equal motion is defined within the framework of perspective—it includes all motions on tracks that converge to a common vanishing point on the picture plane.

Johansson's analysis of unequal motion vectors can be illustrated with two vectors. The larger vector is assumed to be the sum of two vector components, a portion equal to the other (smaller) vector and a residual. If the two equal vectors are in the same direction, they are processed together to produce perceived rigid motion in the frontal plane; if they are in different directions, they produce perceived rigid motion in depth. The residual vector enters the processing to produce different kinds of responses depending on other aspects of stimulation. It can result in the perception of form change, of perceived rigid rotation in depth, or a combination of rotary motion and form change. For Johansson, the perceptual system analyzes the changing proximal stimulus to produce perceptions containing the maximal degree of rigidity in coherent patterns. What is critical for perceiving rigidity is the processing of equal motion components extracted from the proximal stimulus, not whether the distal objects are rigid. This processing is automatic and independent of cognitive control.

Johansson proposed that the perceived object is the simplest possible geometrical object whose distal motion could have produced the proximal stimulus. This *minimum principle* suggests that perception of objects of constant form moving in 3D space is "preferred" over 2D form change. Thus, if the proximal pattern corresponds to the projection of such an object, a moving rigid object is perceived. That is, perceived size and shape constancy are consequences of perceived rigidity and, therefore, are obtained automatically (Cutting & Proffitt, 1982; Hatfield & Epstein, 1985; Hochberg, 1957; Johansson, 1964).

Unity Principle

The demonstration that perceptions tend to be organized or unified can be described as a *unity principle*. Figure 12.4 shows how Johansson demonstrated his vector analysis and the operation of a unity principle using the motion of three vertically aligned dots. The distal motions of the dots are congruent with their proximal motions because the stimulus is in the frontal plane. The lefthand portion of the figure illustrates the proximal motion of the dots: The upper and lower dots *(A and C)* oscillate from left to right, and the middle dot *(B)* oscillates diagonally from lower left to upper right. The motions are synchronized so that the dots remain aligned vertically.

The middle portion of the figure illustrates the perceptual outcome: The three dots appear to oscillate horizontally in synchrony and, simultaneously, the middle dot appears to oscillate vertically. Moreover, the three dots appear to be part of a single unit or object oscillating from left to right. The righthand portion of the figure illustrates Johansson's vector analysis. The diagonal proximal motion of the middle dot is analyzed into horizontal and vertical components: The horizontal vector component is equal in magnitude and direction to the motion vectors of the other dots. This produces the unity in the perceptual outcome. The vertical vector component is the residual and corresponds to the perceived vertical motion of the dot within the unit. Thus, according to Johansson, the perceptual vector analysis explains why dot *B* appears to move up and down vertically within the perceived unified object as the object moves back and forth from left to right.

Rigidity Principle

A *rigidity principle* describes the fact that perceptions tend to be organized as motions of rigid objects in 3D space. Johansson demonstrated the operation

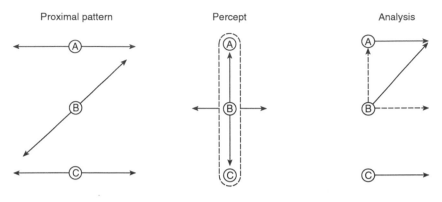

Figure 12.4
Johansson's demonstration of the unity principle and vector analysis. The proximal pattern on the left is perceived as a single object moving laterally (center). Dot *B* appears to move up and down vertically within the object and laterally within the object defined by dots *A* and *C*.

of a rigidity principle in an experiment using the motion of dots following circular or elliptical paths. Figure 12.5 illustrates the different proximal patterns that he used and their perceptual outcomes. The first example in figure 12.5a shows a single dot moving in a circular path on an oscilloscope screen. Once again, the distal motions of the dots are in the frontal plane and, therefore, are congruent with their proximal motions. The perception produced by this stimulus is also illustrated in the figure. Subjects reported seeing a single dot moving in a circular path in the frontal plane.

The second stimulus, figure 12.5b contains a pair of dots moving in the same circular path and positioned at opposite ends of a diameter. Subjects reported that the dots appeared to be connected by a rigid rod rotating in the frontal plane. Thus, the mere presence of a second dot resulted in an apparent connection between the dots (the unity principle) and, in addition, the connection appeared to be rigid (the rigidity principle). In the third stimulus, figure 12.5c, the path was changed to an ellipse. Once again the dots appeared to be the endpoints of a rigid rod, but the rod appeared to rotate in a plane slanted in depth with respect to the viewer. In this example, the organization of the percept as a rigid object forced the perceived motion into the third dimension.

Common and Relative Vectors
The vector ideas of Johansson provided the foundation for the work of Börjesson and von Hofsten (1972, 1973, 1975, 1977) on the perceived

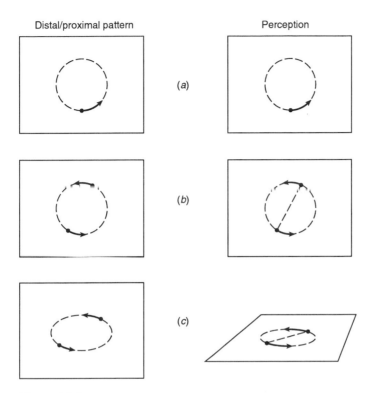

Figure 12.5
Patterns used by Johansson to illustrate the rigidity principle. (a) A single moving dot is perceived as it is. (b) Dots at opposite positions in a circular motion pattern appear to be connected by an invisible rigid rodlike object. (c) Two dots at opposite positions in an elliptical path also appear to be connected by an invisible rigid rod, but the circular motion appears to be in a surface slanted in depth.

motions of two and three points. They defined *common motion vectors* as the proximal motions of two points that are equal in direction and magnitude. They defined *relative motion vectors* as the proximal motions of two points that are equal in magnitude but opposite in direction. The idea was to explain all possible perceived motions as combinations of two simple proximal motion vectors.

The eight possible combinations of common and relative motion are illustrated in figure 12.6. Börjesson and von Hofsten (1972) tested their hypothesis in a series of experiments using two moving dots. Common motion alone (boxes 2 and 3) produced the perception of motion in the frontal plane. Collinear relative motion with no common motion (box 4), and combined with collinear common motion (box 5), were ambiguous

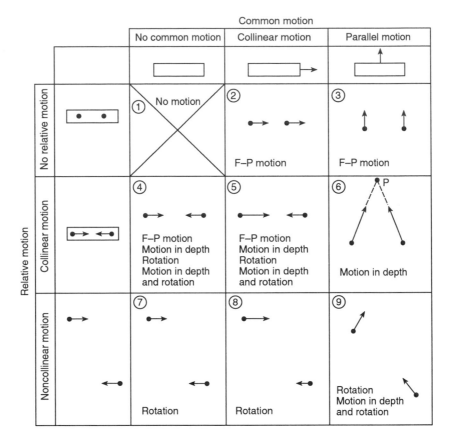

Figure 12.6
Börjesson and von Hofsten's (1972, 1973) analysis of common and relative proximal
motion vectors. Perceptual outcomes are described within each box (see text for
details).

stimuli. Subjects reported all possible perceptions: motion in the frontal
plane, radial motion in depth, rotation in depth, and a combination of radial
motion and rotation in depth. In contrast, collinear relative motion combined with parallel motion (box 6) was one of the most stable stimuli—it
produced the perception of motion in depth. Noncollinear relative motion
alone (box 7), and combined with collinear common motion (box 8), were
also stable—they produced the perception of rotation in depth. Noncollinear relative motion combined with parallel common motion (box 9)
produced the perception of rotation in depth or rotation and radial motion
in depth.

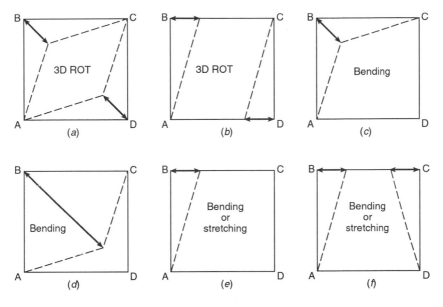

Figure 12.7
Stimuli used by Jansson and Johansson (1973) to study nonrigid perceptions such as bending, folding, and stretching.

Nonrigid Perceptions: Bending, Folding, and Stretching

Nonrigid perceptions such as bending, folding, and stretching have been studied by Johansson and his coworkers (Jansson & Johansson, 1973; Jansson & Runeson, 1977). Figure 12.7 shows the six stimuli used by Jansson and Johansson (1973). The distal 2D motion patterns were presented in a frontal plane and, therefore, are congruent with the proximal motion patterns. In each pattern, a square changed into one of six other shapes produced by motion of one or two of the corners.

Thirty subjects described the motion patterns as rotation, bending, or stretching, and could add verbal descriptions if desired. *Perceived rotation* was defined as a plane object, possibly rigid, that moves in rotary motion in 3D space. The object could change form and/or size to some extent. *Perceived bending* was defined in two ways: It could describe the gradual deformation of a rectangular piece of paper when two opposite corners bend toward each other, or the folding of two rigid plane surfaces about a common axis ("bookfolding"). In both of these perceptions, the properties of the object remain unchanged. The essential difference is that the components are rigid in one aspect and nonrigid in the other. *Perceived stretching* involves deformation of the surface such as that resulting from pulling on a rubber sheet.

In stimulus *(a)*, opposite corners moved back and forth along the diagonal and, in *(b)*, they moved toward an adjacent corner. These patterns were described primarily as perceived rotation in 3D (by 97% and 87% of the subjects, respectively). In stimulus *(c)*, a corner moved one-quarter of the way along the diagonal and, in *(d)*, it moved three-quarters of the way. These patterns were described primarily as perceived bending (by 97% and 83% of the subjects, respectively). The responses were less stable when a single corner moved along a side toward an adjacent corner as in *(e)*, or when two adjacent corners moved along a side toward each other as in *(f)*. These motions were described as perceived bending and stretching (63% and 33% for the former and 40% and 43% for the latter, respectively).

Jansson and Johansson (1973) explained the outcomes of the experiment by extending the minimum principle to include partially rigid motions such as bending. Thus, they suggested, rotation was the preferred perception when rotation of an approximately rigid surface was geometrically possible. For example, when two opposite corners of a square moved, rotation of an approximately rigid surface was possible geometrically and, therefore, rotation was the predominant response.

Computation or Artificial Intelligence Approach

Computational theories about perceived rotary motion focus on the *structure-from-motion* problem, how to compute 3D rigid-object rotation from motion patterns in the proximal stimulus (see Braunstein, 1962, 1976; Johansson, 1978a, 1978b; Johansson, von Hofsten, & Jansson, 1980; Todd, 1985; Ullman, 1979a, for reviews). Some of the theories consist of algorithms that can be used in artificial intelligence devices (computers) that have important practical applications such as military target identification.

Many computational analyses construct a unique 3D "interpretation" of the 2D input based on the *rigidity assumption,* the assumption that the proximal stimulus was produced by a rigid distal object (Todd, 1982, 1984, 1985; Ullman, 1979a, 1979b). Although this assumption does fairly well with rigid perceptions, it has difficulties explaining nonrigid perceptions such as bending, stretching, and shrinking. One way around this difficulty is to invoke an executive or preprocessor that controls a sequence of tests.

The first test determines whether the proximal pattern has a possible rigid interpretation. If it does not, a different algorithm is applied, one that is appropriate for nonrigid motion (Lee, 1974; Todd, 1982; Ullman, 1979a, 1979b).

Structure-from-motion algorithms must also solve the *correspondence problem,* the ability to identify and keep track of stimulus points that correspond over time (Todd, 1985). The problem arises from the fact that the proximal input is a moving 2D pattern whose elements change position over time. The visual system must be able to identify and keep track of individual points as they move over time (Marr & Poggio, 1976, Ullman, 1979a, 1979b). In a sense, this problem is analogous to the identification of corresponding points in stereopsis (chapter 3; Julesz, 1971; Longuet-Higgins & Prazdny, 1980). The correspondence problem is difficult because there are situations in which elements in the proximal stimulus do not persist over time (Todd, 1985; Ullman, 1979a). Occlusion is, perhaps, the most important example: Near objects occlude portions of more distant objects and there is continuous disappearance and reappearance of points when motion is introduced (see section on dynamic occlusion in chapter 10).

Patterns of Deformation: Differential Invariants of Optic Flow

The optic array undergoes deformation when the viewer moves, or when objects move in the environment. These motions are manifested in two types of local features of the optical flow—average flow velocity at a particular location and the structure of the local variation of velocity in the immediate neighborhood of the locality. The latter, the *local parallax field,* can be described by deformation analysis.

Koenderink and van Doorn (1975, 1976, 1981; Koenderink, 1985, 1986) proposed that the motion parallax field can be specified by three differential invariants of the optic flow (divergence, vorticity, and deformation or shear) and a given direction (the axis of dilation of the shear), all of which vary as a function of position and time. Deformations can be measured (over time) relative to the previous image. Therefore coordinates are not needed. The proposed invariants are illustrated in figure 12.8. *Divergence* describes a homogeneous stretch, i.e., a magnification (expansion) or minification (contraction) of a pattern without change of shape. It is numerically equal to the relative rate of change of the solid angle. *Vorticity* describes a rigid rotation (the rate of rotation is the *curl*). *Deformation* or *shear*

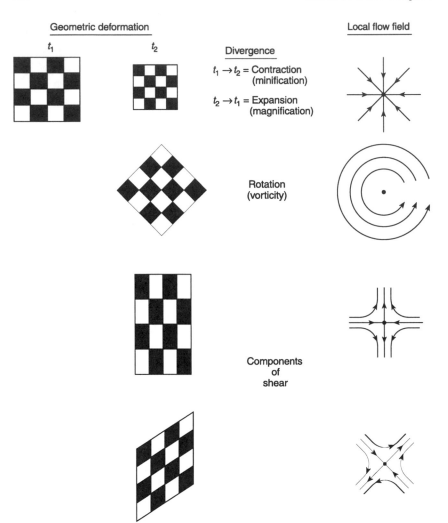

Figure 12.8
Geometrical deformations of optical flow and vector patterns of the local flow field
described by Koenderink and van Doorn (1975, 1976, 1981; Koenderink, 1985,
1986).

describes an expansion in one direction accompanied by a contraction in an orthogonal direction such that solid angle is conserved. Shear alters the orientation of small elements in the optic array but there is no rotation. The axis of dilation of the shear must also be specified.

The identification of invariants in the optic flow field implies that processing algorithms respond to the invariants to produce corresponding perceptions. For example, Longuet-Higgins and Prazdny (1980) demonstrated that, in principle, the instantaneous retinal velocity field determines the structure of the rigid scene and the direction of motion. Their analysis of the optic flow field produced by a rigid, textured, curved surface resulted in a vector sum of translational and rotational components. The translational velocity at any point is directed toward or away from a unique vanishing point determined by the relative translational motion, and the relational velocity field is determined by the angular velocity of the eye relative to the environment. These components can be calculated using the information in motion parallax. Longuet-Higgins and Prazdny concluded that second derivatives are needed in addition to the differential invariants described by Koenderink and van Doorn (1976) for a full determination of the relative motion of the observer.

There is an important difference, however, between a psychological theory and artificial intelligence computations that solve specific detection problems. Psychological theory attempts to describe visual system processing, whereas computational algorithms describe possible ways to solve specific problems. Consequently, in evaluating whether a specific computational theory is also a viable psychological explanation, one must assess the degree to which it provides a plausible account of visual system processing. If it does, the assumptions associated with the computation may describe constraints by which the visual system functions. If it does not, the computation may be best suited for machine vision applications, having little in common with actual perceptual processes (Todd, 1985). In one evaluation, Todd (1984) tested the psychological validity of various computational analyses by determining whether their assumptions imposed limitations consistent with those of actual human observers. He found that existing algorithms probably have little in common with processes of the human visual system. This finding underscores the importance of testing computational proposals against actual perceptual system performance.

Summary

The rotating trapezoidal illusion, the kinetic depth effect, and the stereo-kinetic effect show the importance of a changing proximal pattern for producing the perception of rigid object motions. Johansson explained visual motion perception using a vector analysis and automatic application of unity, rigidity, and minimum principles. Computational and artificial intelligence approaches define higher-order mathematical properties of the proximal motion pattern.

13

Detecting Motion

The preceding three chapters discussed the perception of moving objects and motion of the perceiver. The focus of this chapter is motion detection. The discussion of detecting motion is divided into two components: stimulus analysis and model construction.

In the context of detection, *stimulus analysis* implies more than the analysis of complex stimuli into motion components (as described in previous chapters). In this chapter, the focus is on psychophysical experiments that isolate stimulus patterns that elicit responses from "detectors," hypothetical structures in the visual system. This analysis follows the conception of Lettvin, Maturana, McCulloch, and Pitts (1959; Lettvin, Maturana, Pitts, & McCulloch, 1961), who found structural units in the visual system (retina) of the frog that respond directly to specific complex properties of stimulation.

The second aspect of discussing detection follows Reichardt (1957, 1961) by describing models of units that could achieve the motion analysis. Reichardt's (1957, 1961) model was the first computational (and structural) model. Although it was developed to explain the response of insects to relative movement of the optical surroundings, it has been adapted for human perception (van Santen & Sperling, 1984). The chapter begins by describing a simple linear motion detector based on this model and continues with the discussion of different complex global patterns.

Motion in the Frontal Plane

Motion detectors are conceptual models of structural units in the visual system that respond to a specific proximal motion pattern, i.e., the detectors are "tuned" to a single specific pattern of proximal motion (Lu & Sperling,

1995, 1996; Nakayama, 1985; Regan, 1986b; Reichardt, 1957, 1961; Sekuler, 1975; Sekuler, Pantle, & Levinson, 1978). For example, a motion detector may respond to a contour moving across the visual field in a specific proximal meridian or orientation. Figure 13.1 shows two simple patterns typically used to stimulate motion detectors: *(a)* a single contour and *(b)* a *grating,* a regular pattern of alternating stripes, moving in a direction that is orthogonal to the orientation of the contours.

Psychophysical studies that provide evidence for the existence of motion detectors compare responses to different stimulus patterns. Two visual responses have been used frequently: the motion aftereffect and the threshold for detecting motion. A *motion aftereffect (MAE)* is produced by fixating a moving stimulus for a period of time, then replacing it with a test stimulus, a stationary contour or grating, that is similar to the original. The stationary stimulus will appear to move in a direction opposite to that of the original motion. The perceived aftereffect motion will be relatively strong at first but will weaken rapidly and disappear. The decay of the *MAE* is indexed by a *decay time constant,* the time it takes for the strength of the aftereffect to fall to $1/e$ (approximately one-third) of its initial value.

The threshold for the detection of motion is the point on a stimulus dimension below which perceived motion is not reported and above which perceived motion is reported. Empirically, this conceptual point can only be determined as a proportion of responses of a particular sort (typically, 75 percent reported motion). Elevation of the threshold for detecting motion, *detection threshold elevation (DTE),* is a measure of the amount by which

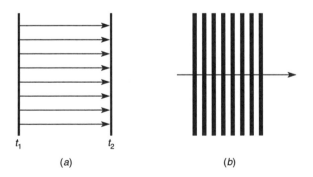

t_1 t_2

(a)   (b)

Figure 13.1
Two simple patterns that stimulate motion detectors: (a) a single moving contour and (b) a moving grating. The motion is orthogonal to the orientation of the contour or grating.

stimulus motion must be increased, i.e., made faster or more intense, for the viewer to detect it. The idea is that, after viewing oscillatory motion over a specific area of the visual field, the ability to detect motion is reduced, so that the threshold for detecting motion is raised.

Linear Motion Detector

Figure 13.2 shows a conceptual model of a motion detector. In Figure 13.2a, the stimulus is illustrated as if looking into the eye. A vertical contour moves horizontally across the visual field to stimulate discrete receptor units A at t_1 and B at t_2. These are schematic representations and each unit may consist of a network of cells in the visual system.

Figure 13.2b shows a schematic representation of the logical interconnections of a structure that could produce a signal whose output is the detection of motion. The component MD represents an integrating unit that responds only when it receives asynchronous input from A and B. Receptor unit A, stimulated at t_1, sends a signal to MD. The signal can be

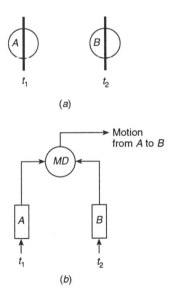

(a)

(b)

Figure 13.2
(a) A vertical contour moves horizontally across the visual field, stimulating discrete receptor units in the visual system, A at t_1 and B at t_2, represented in the figure as if looking into the eye at the receptor surface. (b) A motion detector: a hypothetical structure whose output signals the detection of motion from position A to position B over time interval t_1 to t_2.

delayed, as in Reichardt's (1957, 1961; van Santen & Sperling, 1984) conception, or it may be below the threshold for response and stored by *MD*. In either case, *MD* does not respond. Receptor unit *B* sends a signal to *MD* at t_2. In Reichardt's conception, the delayed signal from *A* and the signal from *B* arrive at *MD* at the same time, triggering a response. In the alternative conception, the signal from *B* adds to the stored subthreshold signal from *A* to produce a signal that is above threshold, and *MD* responds. In either case, the response of *MD* can be interpreted as a signal for the detection of motion in the frontal plane from *A* to *B* over time interval t_1 to t_2.

Thus, the motion detector may be taken as a model of a unit in the visual system that responds directly to local motion in the proximal stimulus. However, it is clear from figure 13.2 that the model does not require continuous motion. The motion detector can operate in response to the stimulus sequence: Stimulate receptor unit *A* at t_1 and unit *B* at t_2. It does not require a stimulus that moves across the field from *A* to *B*. This stimulus sequence is the stimulus for the perception of apparent motion (see chapter 7).

Occluded Motion: The Aperture Problem

Despite the usefulness of the motion detector model, there are a number of situations in which it does not appear adequate. For example, the perception of motion through an aperture suggests that additional analyses may be required. The *aperture problem* posed by a grating moving behind a circular aperture (Wallach, 1935) is illustrated in figure 13.3a). The grating may move in many different directions; however, the perceived direction of motion is usually orthogonal to the orientation of the stripes. Thus, a simple local reading of direction or velocity is not enough information to specify a unique perception corresponding to the actual direction of motion of the grating. This perceptual outcome suggests that perception of the direction of motion is not a direct outcome of action of local motion detectors.

Some factors that might be involved are illustrated by the *barber pole effect* produced by a rectangular aperture (Wallach, 1935). In figure 13.3b, the direction of perceived motion corresponds to the long dimension of the aperture. Hildreth (1984) and Nakayama and Silverman (1985) suggested that the number of line terminations at the edges of apertures determine the perceived direction of motion. Because the vertical aperture has more

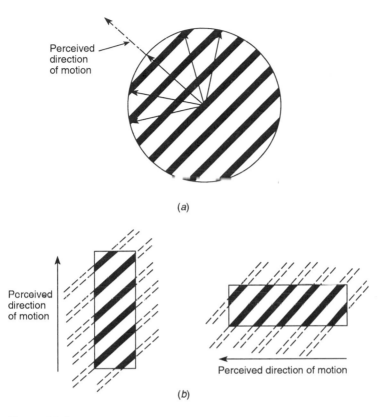

(a)

(b)

Figure 13.3
(a) The *aperture problem:* A grating moving behind a circular aperture could be moving in different directions. The perceived direction is usually orthogonal to the orientation of the stripes. (b) The *barber pole effect:* With rectangular apertures, the direction of perceived motion usually corresponds to the long dimension of the aperture.

terminators moving vertically, the lines appear to be part of a rigid surface moving in the direction of the majority of line terminators.

Occluded Motion: Movement-Dependent Subjective Contours
The perception of movement-dependent subjective contours also raises questions about the adequacy of a local-motion-detector explanation of perceived motion. Recall that subjective contours are contours that appear in areas of the visual field where no stimulus exists. Tynan and Sekuler (1975) produced subjective contours by covering the center portion of a horizontally moving vertical grating with a horizontal strip of black tape.

The interrupted vertical contours appeared to be joined by faint moving subjective contours. However, unlike static subjective contours, these contours were not seen when the grating was stationary, i.e., they depended on stimulus motion.

Weisstein, Maguire, and Berbaum (1977) showed, moreover, that these subjective moving contours gave rise to *MAEs*. Using a similar display, they stopped the motion and removed the tape, exposing the stationary grating. Now, an *MAE* was reported—the stationary contours in the area that was previously covered appeared to move in the opposite direction.

Weisstein and Maguire (1978) showed that the perceived depth relation between the moving grating and the occluding opaque region was crucial for seeing the subjective contours. When the opaque region appeared to be in front of the grating (closer to the observer), the contours were not seen. When it appeared to be in the same plane as the grating or behind it, the contours were visible. The relationship worked both ways: apparent depth affected the illusion and the illusion affected the apparent depth. Thus, Weisstein and her colleagues argued that the perception of subjective contours and *MAEs* cannot be accounted for solely in terms of local (retinal) interactions (Weisstein, Maguire, & Williams, 1982).

Size-Change Detector

A size-change stimulus was described previously as a 1D change in visual angle or proximal size. However, size-change also describes a change in solid visual angle if the change takes place in only a single meridian. Such a pattern is illustrated in figure 13.4 for both decreasing and increasing proximal size-change patterns. The figure shows a pair of parallel contours

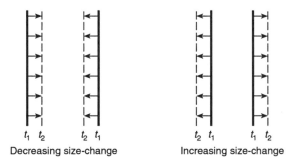

Figure 13.4
Decreasing and increasing size-change patterns produced by the motion of contours.

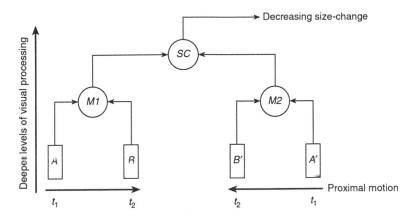

Figure 13.5
A schematic representation of a size–change detector illustrating hierarchical processing. The two motion detectors *(M1* and *M2)* detect motion in opposite directions
and stimulate an integrative unit *(SC)* whose output signals size-change.

that move toward (left side) or away from (right side) each other over time
interval t_1 to t_2.

A schematic model for a size-change detector is presented in figure
13.5. This model represents a conceptualization of structural units in the
visual system that respond specifically to proximal size change. The model
illustrated is a hierarchical model based on the ideas of Regan and Beverley
(1978a, 1978b, 1980; Beverley & Regan, 1979). The lowest level shows
two linear motion detectors *(M1* and *M2)* that respond only to motion in
opposite directions over the same time interval. The outputs of these motion
detectors feed a higher-level integrator *(SC)*. The directions of sensitivity
indicated for the motion detectors are specific to the detectors and are
essential for the construction of the higher-level structure. The output of
the higher unit signals decreasing size-change from *A-A'* to *B-B'*, over time
interval t_1 to t_2.

This model is a hierarchical processing model. It suggests that deeper
levels of the visual system automatically integrate information from different
parts of the visual field. The consequence is that the output of these higher
units can have a new meaning, an emergent meaning that is not evident in
the stimulation or in the output of the lower levels. Models of this sort are
doubly important—they not only provide explanations for specific perceptual phenomena; they also provide a conceptual basis for more complex
theories of direct perceptions. That is, if a prewired structure can respond
to a global stimulus pattern such as size-change, other prewired structures

might exist that respond to more complex stimulus patterns such as the differential invariants described in chapter 12 and below.

Expansion/Contraction or Motion-in-Depth Detector

An increasing or decreasing solid visual angle that changes in more than a single meridian is a proximal (optical) *expansion* or *contraction pattern* (see chapter 11 and figure 11.4). Figure 13.6 shows a conceptual model of an *(E/C)* detector following the ideas of Regan and Beverley (1978a, 1978b; Beverley & Regan, 1979). This is a simplified conceptual model of a structural unit in the visual system that responds specifically to expansion or contraction in the proximal stimulus.

At the lowest levels, there are four motion detectors *(M1, M2, M3, and M4)*. Each detector responds when stimulated by a specific direction of

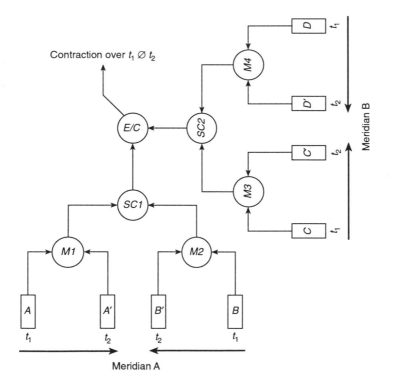

Figure 13.6
A schematic representation of an expansion/contraction detector. Two size-change detectors are oriented in different meridians. They signal decreasing size-change to an integrative unit whose output signals contraction.

motion. At the next higher level, these motion detectors are organized into units that respond to size-change in two different meridians *(SC1* and *SC2)*. The highest level structure *(E/C)* integrates the information from the two size-change detectors. The output of this system signals expansion (or contraction) from position *ABCD* to position *A'B'C'D'*, over time interval t_1 to t_2 (or vice versa). Because an *E/C* pattern is produced by objects moving in depth, Regan and Beverley called this detector a *motion-in-depth* or *looming* detector.

Deformation Analysis and Detectors

Analysis of the optical flow in terms of differential invariants suggests mechanisms that could monitor these aspects of the flow field. These mechanisms are based on image deformation, i.e., they monitor changes in the geometrical structure of local features in the optic array (see chapter 12). The outputs from simple linear (unidirectional) motion detectors can be combined in different ways to produce mechanisms that could detect these invariants. The possibilities suggested by Koenderink and van Doorn (1976; Koenderink, 1985, 1986) and Longuet-Higgins and Prazdny (1980) are illustrated in figure 13.7. The flow field components are dilation, vorticity, and two components of shear (see figure 12.8).

Psychophysical Evidence for Detectors

In many cases, the evidence for the existence of specific detectors involves determining whether the observed response could have been produced by simple summation of responses to linear motion. If not, it is possible to postulate the existence of a mechanism that processes higher-order stimuli directly.

Linear versus Expansion/Contraction

Figure 13.8 shows the two motion patterns used by Regan and Beverley (1978b) to demonstrate the difference between linear and *E/C* detectors. In the stimulus depicted on the left side of the figure, the opposite edges of the square moved in the same direction (inphase). When the sides of this square oscillated, the fixed-size square oscillated in the frontal plane along the diagonal. In the stimulus depicted on the right side of the figure, the opposite edges of the square moved in opposite directions (in antiphase)

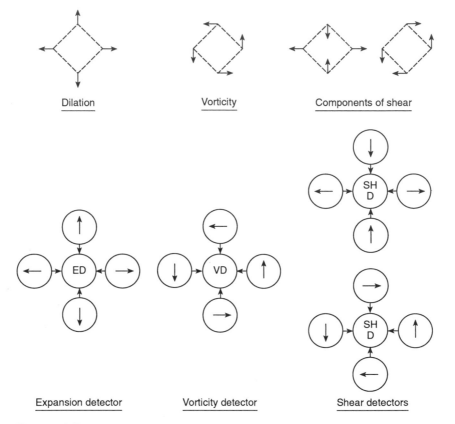

Figure 13.7
Vector patterns for differential invariants of deformation are illustrated in the upper portion (after Longuet-Higgins & Prazdny, 1980). Possible organizations of detector units that could respond to these invariants are illustrated in the lower portion (after Koenderink, 1985, 1986; Koenderink & van Doorn, 1976).

producing an *E/C* pattern. When the sides of this square oscillated, the fixed-position square changed in proximal size.

In the experiment, two identical moving squares were presented on opposite sides of a fixation point so that the eye could not track their motion as the sides oscillated. The two types of motion patterns were presented separately in the same positions so that the sides of the squares oscillated over the exact same retinal regions. Thus, the only difference between the two patterns was the phase of the motion of opposite sides. Consequently, in order to detect the difference in phase, it would be necessary to compare the motion from opposite sides of the square, i.e., from two separate regions of the visual field.

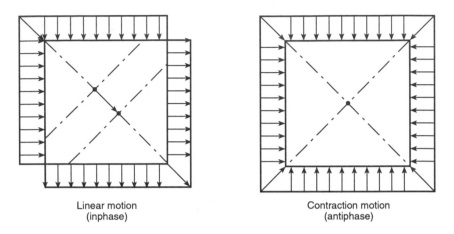

Linear motion
(inphase)

Contraction motion
(antiphase)

Figure 13.8
Stimuli used by Regan and Beverley (1978b) to test for the independence of linear and expansion/contraction (looming) detectors. The stimulus on the left was produced by inphase oscillation and that on the right by antiphase oscillation over the same retinal areas.

If the visual system responds only to *local* stimulation (via unconnected linear motion detectors), the phase difference would not be detected and there would be no differences in the responses to the two patterns. If, however, the phase difference does produce differences in the responses, then it could be assumed that the visual system contains a mechanism for responding directly to a comparison of the stimulus motion from two separated regions of the visual field.

Regan and Beverley (1978b) measured the relative loss in sensitivity to motion after viewing each stimulus. The difference in DTE was large, supporting the claim that the different responses were mediated by different structures in the visual system. This finding is evidence for a structure in the visual system that integrates information from separated parts of the visual field. Not only were the $DTEs$ different for the two types of stimuli, but subjects viewing the antiphase stimulus reported a qualitative difference—the linear stimulus appeared to be a square moving in the frontal plane whereas the antiphase stimulus appeared to be a square moving in depth. Therefore, Regan and Beverley (1980) called the visual mechanism a *looming* detector.

Size-Change versus Expansion/Contraction

To determine whether a proximal E/C pattern is different from a simple size-change pattern, Beverley and Regan (1979) produced motion

aftereffects using the stimulus illustrated in figure 13.9. Two vertical contours moved horizontally within a horizontal band of light. That is, the distance between the contours changed in size in a single proximal meridian. There were two stimulus patterns: The contours moved toward or away from each other over the interval t_1 to t_2 and, instantaneously, appeared back at their original positions and moved again. This cycling, called a *ramping motion,* was repeated during the adapting period. When the motion stopped, subjects reported a size-change *MAE* of the increasing or decreasing size-change for the pattern.

Beverley and Regan (1979) concluded that there is a size-change detector that is different from a linear motion detector. Furthermore, subjects reported that, when this *MAE* dissipated, they experienced a longer-lasting motion-in-depth *MAE*. Regan and Beverley explained this finding as the output of two different levels of a hierarchically arranged detector system—the higher the level, the longer it takes for the aftereffect to decay. They proposed, therefore, that this evidence supported the existence of an *E/C* detector at a processing level different from a size-change detector.

Independence of Expansion/Contraction Detector

Antiphase oscillation of the sides of the proximal square pattern in figure 13.8 produced the perception of a square moving in depth (motion along z-axis). When the sides oscillated in phase, the square appeared to move in the frontal plane—oscillation of the vertical sides produced per-

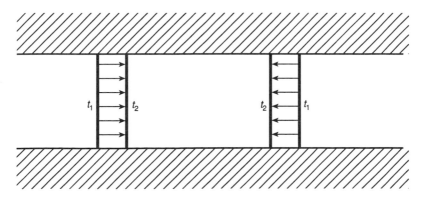

Figure 13.9
Stimulus used by Regan and Beverley (1979) to test for the independence of size-change and expansion/contraction detectors.

ceived sideways or lateral motion (i.e., motion along the x-axis) and oscillation of the horizontal sides produced perceived vertical motion (i.e., motion along the y-axis).

Regan and Beverley (1980) combined an antiphase oscillation (E/C) with an inphase x-axis oscillation to produce the perception of a small (0.5 deg) square stimulus moving in depth at an angle to the viewer. That is, the square appeared to move simultaneously in depth and laterally across the visual field. They used a single antiphase pattern combined with 11 different inphase patterns to produce 11 different trajectories. Thresholds were measured for pure inphase (lateral motion) and pure antiphase (E/C) motion. Threshold elevation to the inphase oscillations increased progressively with the increase in amplitude of the inphase component. However, threshold elevation to the antiphase component remained at the same level throughout, i.e., it was independent of the amount of inphase motion added to the stimulus. Regan and Beverley (1980) concluded that the visual channels that detect the E/C component of proximal stimulus motion are independent of the channels that detect motion in the frontal plane.

A similar result was obtained from measurements of the rotational, radial, and motion-in-depth *MAEs* produced by rotating spirals (Hershenson, 1987). The physical motion of a spiral is measured by vectors normal to the spiral at each point. The relative sizes of the radial and rotational components of this vector are determined by the length of the spiral. Therefore, differences in the length of the spiral arms predict differences in the relative strengths of the rotational and radial *MAEs*. Furthermore, as the spiral rotates, there is radial motion in all directions, producing a stimulus equivalent to an E/C pattern. Therefore, this stimulus produces both radial (E/C) and motion-in-depth *MAEs*.

MAEs were obtained over spokes and concentric circle patterns, i.e., test stimuli orthogonal to the direction of motion of the rotational and radial vector components, respectively. A floating disc test stimulus elicited the motion-in-depth *MAE*. The relative strength of the rotational and radial (E/C) *MAEs* were predicted by the relative size of the rotational and radial motion components of the spiral arms. The relative strength of the motion-in-depth *MAE* was also predicted by the size of the radial vector. These findings support the notion that the visual system responded to rotational and E/C components of motion rather than to the actual motion described by the normal vector.

Linear versus Rotation

Rotation detectors are conceptual models of structural units in the visual system that respond specifically to rotary motion in the proximal stimulus. Regan and Beverley (1985) found evidence for rotation detectors using the stimuli depicted in figure 13.10. The random-dot pattern in each quadrant moved linearly in the directions shown by the arrows so that one global stimulus had a rotary component but the other did not. *DTE* was measured with a field of rotating random dots. Regan and Beverley (1985) found that the two motion patterns produced differences in *DTE*. Therefore, they concluded that the visual system contains global rotation detectors that are different from simple linear motion detectors. However, the existence of rotation detectors remains in question because results from *MAE* studies (Hershenson, 1993a) and from physiological studies using single-cell recording in monkeys (Tanaka & Saito, 1989) do not support this conclusion.

Direction of Stereomotion in Depth and the V_L/V_R Ratio

Beverley and Regan (1973) measured the threshold amplitudes of disparity oscillations as a function of the ratio of the velocities in the left and right proximal patterns (V_L/V_R). They found different functions for motion directed to the right and to the left. That is, adaptation for motion in depth along a line passing to the left of the nose reduced sensitivity to all trajectories passing to the left. However, sensitivities for trajectories passing to the right were unaffected. Thus, adaptation to the motion-in-depth stimuli was direction-specific, affecting a limited range of V_L/V_R ratios. Beverley and Regan (1973) proposed that, for a given viewing distance, the ratio of the velocities in the left and right proximal patterns (V_L/V_R) determines the direction of perceived object motion in visual space. They concluded that

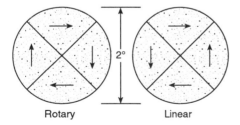

Rotary   Linear

Figure 13.10
Stimulus used by Regan and Beverley (1985) to test for a rotation detector. The random-dot patterns move linearly in the direction of the arrows. The pattern on the left contains a rotation component whereas the pattern on the right does not.

the visual system contains at least two binocular channels for processing proximal trajectories in the two eyes to produce perceived motion in depth.

Summary

Motion detectors are conceptual models of units in the visual system that respond to a specific proximal pattern. Detectors have been proposed for detecting linear motion, size-change, expansion/contraction, and rotation in the proximal stimulus. Psychophysical evidence from studies of *MAEs* and thresholds supports most of these proposals.

14

Concluding Thoughts

What can be said about the wonderful system that produces our awareness of visual space? This chapter presents some concluding generalities that have been repeatedly demonstrated over the course of describing the operation of that system.

There are a number of generalizations that provide the foundation for the understanding of visual space perception. First, the proximal stimulus is important and the distal stimulus is not. Second, perception is emergent, i.e., it is determined by perceptual system activity, not the distal stimulus or the proximal stimulus. Third, perceptual processing is global, encompassing more than a single limited (local) area of the visual field. Finally, perceptual processing includes automatic processes as well as cognitive and/or acquired processes.

Distal versus Proximal Stimulus

The first generality is that the important aspect of the input is contained in proximal information, not in properties of distal objects or spaces. This seemingly obvious statement must be made explicit because references to properties of distal objects find their way into explanations of perception. One example is the argument that a rigidity assumption is invalid because nonrigid objects can be perceived.

Emergent Quality of Perception

The proposition that perception is emergent is the assertion that the qualities of perception are not determined by the proximal stimulus. They are the result of the activity of the perceptual system. The obvious example is the perception of 3D space and associated perceptual qualities such as solidity and rigidity. But there are many other examples including subjective contours (both binocular and monocular) and figure-ground relations.

Global Aspect of Perception

There is ample evidence throughout the book that perceptual processing is global in nature. This was true in the discussion of retinal disparity and binocular rivalry, in the perception of depth from shadows, in induced and apparent motion, in the aperture problem, and in the detection of expansion/contraction, to name just a few. The implication is not only that there is parallel processing but that the processing is integrated along the way.

Automatic Mechanisms and Cognitive Factors

There is also ample evidence that perceptual processing includes automatic processes as well as cognitive and/or acquired processes. Whether one or the other predominates is not clear at present. As knowledge of brain processes grows, the data appear to be shifting more and more toward automatic processes. Nevertheless, there appears to be a role for experience, at least in coordinating perceptual and motor systems and in scaling the perception of space to the size of our bodies.

Appendix: Angular Measures

Angles are measured in radians (rad) or in degrees of arc (deg). One degree contains 60 minutes of arc (min) and one minute contains 60 seconds of arc (sec). In the text, *deg*, *min*, and *sec* are used for angular measurements of *arc*.

The relationship between radians and degrees is illustrated in figure A.1. In general, if S is the length of the arc subtended at the center of the circle by the angle Θ (rad) and R is the radius of a circle, then $\Theta = S/R$. One *radian* is the angle subtended at the center of a circle by an arc whose length equals the radius of the circle. The circumference of the circle (C) is given by $2\pi R$, where R is the radius and $\pi = 3.1416 \ldots$ Hence, there are 2π or $6.2832 \ldots$ radians in one complete revolution (360 deg) and $1 \text{ rad} = 360/2\pi = 57.3 \ldots$ deg.

The visual angle subtended at the eye by an object is given by the ratio of the size of the object to its distance from the viewer (measured to the nodal point of the eye, approximately 7 mm behind the cornea). For small angles (less than about 10 degrees), $\tan \alpha = \alpha$.

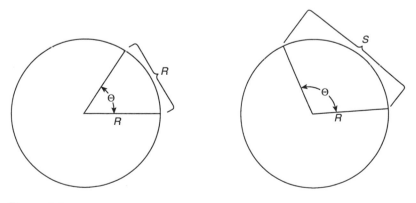

Figure A.1
Measuring angles in radians. In the circle on the left, Θ equals one radian and in the general case, on the right, $\Theta = S/R$ radians.

Table A.1 contains examples of some visual angles subtended by familiar objects. The sun and moon subtend visual angles of about 0.5 deg. Your thumbnail at arm's length is about 1.5 to 2 deg.

Table A.1

Object	Distance	Visual Angle
Sun	93,000,000 mi	0.5 deg
Moon	240,000 mi	0.5 deg
Thumbnail	arm's length	1.5–2 deg
Lowercase letter	reading distance	13 min

References

Abbreviations:

AJP: *American Journal of Psychology*
JEP: *Journal of Experimental Psychology*
JEP:HP&P: *Journal of Experimental Psychology: Human Perception and Performance*
JOSA: *Journal of the Optical Society of America*
PB: *Psychological Bulletin*
P&P: *Perception & Psychophysics*
PR: *Psychological Review*
VR: *Vision Research*

Akerstrom, R. A., & Todd, J. T. (1988). The perception of stereoscopic transparency. *P&P, 44*, 421–432.

Alpern, M. (1962). Introduction to movements of the eyes. In H. Davson (Ed.), *The eye. Vol. 3: Muscular mechanisms* (pp. 3–5). New York: Academic Press.

Ames, A., Jr. (1951). Visual perception and the rotating trapezoidal window. *Psychological Monographs, 65*, No. 324.

Ames, A., Jr. (1955). *An interpretive manual for the demonstrations in the psychology research center.* Princeton, NJ: Princeton University Press.

Andersen, G. J. (1989). Perception of three-dimensional structure from optic flow without locally smooth velocity. *JEP:HP&P, 15*, 363-371.

Arditi, A. (1986). Binocular vision. In K. R. Boff, L. Kaufman, & J. P. Thomas (Eds.), *Handbook of perception and performance. Vol. I: Sensory processes and perception.* New York: Wiley.

Attneave, F. (1954). Some informational aspects of visual perception. *PR, 61*, 183–193.

Attneave, F. (1982). Prägnanz and soap bubble systems: A theoretical exploration. In J. Beck, (Ed.), *Organization and representation in perception* (pp. 11–29). Hillsdale, NJ: Erlbaum.

Attneave, F., & Block, G. (1973). Apparent movement in tridimensional space. *P&P, 13*, 301–307.

Barbeito, R. (1981). Sighting dominance: An explanation based on the processing of visual direction in tests of sighting dominance. *VR, 21*, 855–860.

Barbeito, R. & Ono, H. (1979). Four methods of locating the egocenter: A comparison of their predictive validities and reliabilities. *Behavioral Research Methods and Instrumentation, 11,* 31–36.

Beck, J. (1982). *Organization and representation in perception.* Hillsdale, NJ: Erlbaum.

Beck, J., & Gibson, J. J. (1955). The relation of apparent shape to apparent slant in the perception of objects. *JEP, 50,* 125–133.

Berkeley, G. (1709/1963). An essay toward a new theory of vision. Reprinted in C. M. Turbayne, (Ed.), *Berkeley's works on vision,* New York: Bobbs-Merrill.

Beverley, K. I., & Regan, D. (1973). Evidence for the existence of neural mechanisms selectively sensitive to the direction of movement in space. *Journal of Physiology, 235,* 17–29.

Beverley, K. I., & Regan, D. (1979). Separable aftereffects of changing-size and motion-in-depth: Different neural mechanisms? *VR, 19,* 727–732.

Beverley, K. I., & Regan, D. (1983). Texture changes versus size changes as stimuli for motion in depth. *VR, 12,* 1387–1400.

Blake, R., Fox, R., & Westendorf, D. H. (1974). Visual size constancy occurs after binocular rivalry. *VR, 14,* 585–586.

Blake, R., O'Shea, R. P., & Mueller, T. J. (1991). Spatial zones of binocular rivalry in central and peripheral vision. *Visual Neuroscience, 8,* 469–478.

Bootsma, R. J., & Oudejans, R. R. D. (1993). Visual information about time-to-collision between two objects. *JEP:HP&P, 19,* 1041–1052.

Boring, E. G. (1942). *Sensation and perception in the history of experimental psychology.* New York: Appleton-Century-Crofts.

Börjesson, E., & von Hofsten, C. (1972). Spatial determinants of depth perception in two-dot motion patterns. *P&P, 11,* 263–268.

Börjesson, E., & von Hofsten, C. (1973). Visual perception of motion in depth: Application of a vector analysis to three-dot motion patterns. *P&P, 13,* 169–179.

Börjesson, E., & von Hofsten, C. (1975). A vector model for perceived object rotation and translation in space. *Psychological Research, 38,* 209–230.

Börjesson, E., & von Hofsten, C. (1977). Effects of different motion characteristics on perceived motion in depth. *Scandinavian Journal of Psychology, 18,* 203–208.

Braunstein, M. L. (1962). Perception of depth through motion. *PB, 59,* 422–433.

Braunstein, M. L. (1966). Sensitivity of the observer to transformation of the visual field. *JEP, 72,* 683–689.

Braunstein, M. L. (1968). Motion and texture as sources of slant information. *JEP, 78,* 247-253.

Braunstein, M. L. (1976). *Depth perception through motion.* New York: Academic Press.

Braunstein, M. L., & Tittle, J. S. (1988). The observer-relative velocity field as the basis for effective motion parallax. *JEP:HP&P, 14,* 582–590.

Broerse, J., Ashton, R., & Shaw, C. (1992). The apparent shape of afterimages in the Ames room. *Perception, 21,* 261–268.

Brunswick, E. (1929). Zur Entwicklung der Albedowahrnehmung. *Zeitschrift für Psychologie, 109,* 40–115.

Brunswick, E. (1956). *Perception and the representative design of psychological experiments* (2nd ed.). Berkeley, CA: University of California Press.

Carlson, V. R. (1960). Overestimation in size constancy. *AJP, 73,* 199–213.

Carlson, V. R. (1977). Instructions in perceptual constancy judgments. In W. Epstein, (Ed.), *Stability and constancy in visual perception: Mechanisms and processes* (pp. 217–254). New York: Wiley.

Caudek, C., & Proffitt, D. R. (1993). Depth perception in motion parallax and stereokinesis. *JEP:HP&P, 19,* 32–47.

Cavanagh, P., & Leclerc, Y. G. (1989). Shape from shading. *JEP:HP&P, 15,* 3–27.

Cohen, W. (1957). Spatial and textural characteristics of the *Ganzfeld. AJP, 70,* 403–410.

Collewijn, H., Steinman, R. M., Erkelens, C. J., & Regan, D. (1991). Binocular fusion, stereopsis, and stereoacuity with a moving head. In D. Regan (Ed.), *Vision and visual dysfunction, Vol. 9: Binocular vision* (pp. 121–136). Boca Raton, FL: CRC Press.

Coren, S. (1972). Subjective contours and apparent depth. *PR, 79,* 339–367.

Cormack, R. H. (1984). Stereoscopic depth perception at far viewing distances. *P&P, 35,* 423–428.

Cormack, R., & Fox, R. (1985). The computation of retinal disparity. *P&P, 37,* 176–178.

Cutting, J. E., & Proffitt, D. R. (1982). The minimum principle and the perception of absolute, common, and relative motions. *Cognitive Psychology, 14,* 211–246.

Duncker, K. (1929). Über induzierte Bewegung [On induced motion]. *Psychologische Forschung, 12,* 180–259.

Dwyer, J., Ashton, R., & Broerse, J. (1990). Emmert's law in the Ames room. *Perception, 19,* 35–41.

Ebenholtz, S. M. (1983). Perceptual coding and adaptations of the oculomotor systems. In L. Spillman, & W. Wooten (Eds.), *Sensory experience, adaptation, and perception: Festschrift für Ivo Kohler* (pp. 335–344). Hillsdale, NJ: Erlbaum.

Ebenholtz, S. M. (1988). Long-term endurance of adaptive shifts in tonic accommodation. *Ophthalmic Physiological Optics, 8,* 427–431.

Ebenholtz, S. M. (1991). Accommodative hysteresis: Fundamental asymmetry in decay rate after near and far focusing. *Investigative Ophthalmology & Visual Science, 32,* 148–153.

Ebenholtz, S. M., & Zander, P. A. L. (1987). Accommodative hysteresis: Influence on closed loop measures of far point and near point. *Investigative Ophthalmology & Visual Science, 28,* 1246–1249.

Emmert, E. (1881). Grössenverhältnisse der Nachbilder. *Klinische Monatsblätter für Augenheilkunde, 19,* 443–450.

Enright, J. T. (1989). The eye, the brain, and the size of the moon: Toward a unified oculomotor hypothesis for the moon illusion. In M. Hershenson (Ed.), *The moon illusion* (pp. 59-121). Hillsdale, NJ: Erlbaum.

Epstein, W. (1973). The process of taking-into-account in visual perception. *Perception,* *2,* 267–285.

Epstein, W. (1977a). Historical introduction to the constancies. In W. Epstein (Ed.), *Stability and constancy in visual perception: Mechanisms and processes* (pp. 1–22). New York: Wiley.

Epstein, W. (1977b). *Stability and constancy in visual perception: Mechanisms and processes.* New York: Wiley.

Epstein, W., & Landauer, A. (1969). Size and distance judgments under reduced conditions of viewing. *P&P, 6,* 269–272.

Epstein, W., & Park, J. (1963). Shape constancy: functional relationships and theoretical formulations. *PB, 60,* 265–288.

Epstein, W., Park, J., & Casey, A. (1961). The current status of the size-distance hypothesis. *PB. 58,* 491–514.

Erens, R. G. F., Kappers, A. M., & Koenderink, J. J. (1993a). Estimating local shape from shading in the presence of global shading. *P&P, 54,* 334–342.

Erens, R. G. F., Kappers, A. M., & Koenderink, J. J. (1993b). Perception of local shape from shading. *P&P, 54,* 145–156.

Flock, H. R. (1964a). A possible optical basis for monocular slant perception. *PR, 71,* 380–391.

Flock, H. R. (1964b). Three theoretical views of slant perception. *PB 62,* 110–121.

Foley, J. M. (1966). Locus of perceived equidistance as a function of viewing distance. *JOSA, 56,* 822–827.

Foley, J. M. (1967). Disparity increase with convergence for constant perceptual criteria. *P&P, 2,* 605–609.

Foley, J. M. (1980). Binocular distance perception. *PR, 87,* 411–434.

Foley, J. M. (1991). Binocular space perception. In D. Regan (Ed.), *Vision and visual dysfunction, Vol. 9: Binocular vision* (pp. 75–92). Boca Raton, FL: CRC Press.

Fox, R. (1991). Binocular rivalry. In D. Regan (Ed.), *Vision and visual dysfunction, Vol. 9: Binocular vision* (pp. 93–110). Boca Raton, FL: CRC Press.

Gibson, E. J., Gibson, J. J., Smith, O. W., & Flock, A (1959). Motion parallax as a determinant of perceived depth. *JEP, 54,* 40–51.

Gibson, J. J. (1950a). *The perception of the visual world.* Boston: Houghton Mifflin.

Gibson, J. J. (1950b). The perception of visual surfaces. *AJP, 63,* 367–384.

Gibson, J. J. (1959). Perception as a function of stimulation. In S. Koch (Ed.), *Psychology: A study of a science* (pp. 456–501). New York: McGraw-Hill.

Gibson, J. J. (1966). *The senses considered as perceptual systems.* Boston: Houghton Mifflin.

Gibson, J. J. (1968). What gives rise to the perception of motion? *PR*, *75*, 335–346.

Gibson, J. J. (1979). *The ecological approach to visual perception*. Boston: Houghton Mifflin.

Gibson, J. J., & Carel, W. (1952). Does motion perspective independently produce the impression of a receding surface? *JEP*, *44*, 16–18.

Gibson, J. J., & Gibson, E. J. (1957). Continuous perspective transformations and the perception of rigid motion. *JEP*, *54*, 129–138.

Gibson, J. J., Olum, P., & Rosenblatt, F. (1955). Parallax and perspective during airplane landings. *AJP*, *68*, 372–385.

Gilchrist, A. L. (1977). Perceived lightness depends on perceived spatial arrangement. *Science*, *195*, 185–187.

Gilinsky, A. S. (1951). Perceived size and distance in visual space. *PR*, *58*, 460–482.

Gilinsky, A. S. (1955). The effect of attitude upon the perception of size. *AJP*, *68*, 173–192.

Gilinsky, A. S. (1989). The moon illusion in a unified theory of visual space. In M. Hershenson (Ed.), *The moon illusion* (pp.167–192). Hillsdale, NJ: Erlbaum.

Gogel, W. C. (1965). Equidistance tendency and its consequences. *PB*, *64*, 153–163.

Gogel, W. C. (1969). Equidistance effects in visual fields. *AJP*, *82*, 342–349.

Gogel, W. C. (1977). The metric of visual space. In W. Epstein (Ed.), *Stability and constancy in visual perception: Mechanisms and processes* (pp. 129–181). New York: Wiley.

Gogel, W. C. (1981). The role of suggested size in distance responses. *P&P*, *32*, 241–250.

Gogel, W. C., & Da Silva, J. A. (1987a). Familiar size and the theory of off-sized perceptions. *P&P*, *41*, 318–328.

Gogel, W. C., & Da Silva, J. A. (1987b). A two-process theory of the responses to size and distance. *P&P*, *41*, 220–238.

Gogel, W. C., & Mertz, D. L. (1989). The contribution of heuristic process to the moon illusion. In M. Hershenson, (Ed.), *The moon illusion* (pp. 235–258). Hillsdale, NJ: Erlbaum.

Gogel, W. C., & Teitz, J. D. (1973). Absolute motion parallax and the specific distance tendency. *P&P*, *13*, 284–292.

Graham, C. H. (1951). Visual perception. In S. Stevens (Ed.), *Handbook of experimental psychology* (pp. 868–920). New York: Wiley.

Gruber, H. E. (1954). The relation of perceived size to perceived distance. *AJP*, *67*, 411–426.

Gulick, W. L., & Lawson, R. B. (1976). *Human stereopsis*. New York: Oxford University Press.

Haber, R. N. (1978). Visual perception. In M. R. Rosenzweig & L. W. Porter (Eds.), *Annual Review of Psychology*, *29*, 31–59.

Haber, R. N. (1983). Stimulus information and processing mechanisms in visual space perception. In J. Beck, B. Hope, & A. Rosenfeld (Eds.), *Human and machine vision* (pp. 157–235). New York: Academic Press.

Haber, R. N. (1986). Toward a theory of the perceived layout of scenes. In A. Rosenfeld (Ed.), *Human and machine vision. II* (pp. 109–148). New York: Academic Press.

Haber, R. N., & Hershenson, M. (1980). *The psychology of visual perception.* New York: Holt, Rinehart & Winston.

Harvey, L. O., Jr., & Leibowitz, H. W. (1967). Effects of exposure duration, cue reduction, and temporary monocularity on size matching at short distances. *JOSA, 57,* 249–253.

Hastorf, A. H., & Way, K. S. (1952). Apparent size with and without distance cues. *Journal of General Psychology, 47,* 181–188.

Hatfield, G., & Epstein, W. (1985). The status of the minimum principle in the theoretical analysis of visual perception. *PB, 97,* 155–186.

Helmholtz, H. von (1866/1963). *A treatise on physiological optics (Vol. 3).* (J. P. C. Southall, Ed. & Trans.). New York: Dover.

Henson, D. B. (1993). *Visual fields.* Oxford: Oxford University Press.

Hering, E. (1864). *Beitrage zur Physiologie.* Leipzig: W. Engelman.

Hering, E. (1868/1977). *The theory of binocular vision* (B. Bridgman & L. Stark, Eds. & Trans.). New York: Plenum.

Hershenson, M. (1982). Moon illusion and spiral aftereffect: Illusions due to the loom-zoom system? *JEP: General, 111,* 423–440.

Hershenson, M. (1987). Visual system responds to rotational and size-change components of complex proximal motion patterns. *P&P, 42,* 60-64.

Hershenson, M. (1989a). *The moon illusion.* Hillsdale, NJ: Erlbaum.

Hershenson, M. (1989b). Moon illusion as anomaly. In M. Hershenson (Ed.), *The moon illusion* (pp. 123–145). Hillsdale, NJ: Erlbaum.

Hershenson, M. (1992a). Size-distance invariance: Kinetic invariance is different from static invariance. *P&P, 51,* 541–548.

Hershenson, M. (1992b). The perception of shrinking in apparent motion. *P&P, 52,* 671–675.

Hershenson, M. (1993a). Linear and rotation motion aftereffects as a function of inspection duration. *VR, 33,* 1913–1919.

Hershenson, M. (1993b). Structural constraints: Further evidence from apparent motion in depth. *Perception, 22,* 323–334.

Heuer, H., & Owens, D. A. (1987). Variation in dark vergence as a function of vertical gaze deviation. *Investigative Ophthalmology & Visual Science (Suppl.), 28,* 315.

Heuer, H., Wischmeyer, E., Brüwer, M., & Römer, T. (1991). Apparent size as a function of vertical gaze direction: New tests of an old hypothesis. *JEP:HP&P, 17,* 232–245.

Hildreth, E. C. (1984). *The measurement of visual motion.* Cambridge, MA: MIT Press.

Hillebrand, F. (1893). Die Stabilitat der Raumwerte auf der Netzhaut. *Zeitschrift für Psychologie, 5,* 1–59.

Hochberg, C. B., & Hochberg, J. (1952). Familiar size and the perception of depth. *The Journal of Psychology, 34,* 107–114.

Hochberg, J. (1957). Effects of the *Gestalt* revolution: The Cornell symposium on perception. *PR, 64,* 78–84.

Hochberg, J. (1971). Perception II: Space and movement. In J. W. Kling & L. A. Riggs (Eds.), *Woodworth and Schlosberg's Experimental Psychology* (3rd ed.). New York: Holt, Rinehart & Winston.

Hochberg, J., & Brooks, V. (1960). The psychophysics of form: Reversible-perspective drawings of spatial objects. *AJP, 73,* 337–354.

Hochberg, J. & McAlister, E. (1953). A quantitative approach to figural goodness. *JEP, 46,* 361-364.

Holway, A. H., & Boring, E. G. (1940). The moon illusion and the angle of regard. *AJP, 53,* 109–116.

Holway, A. H., & Boring, E. G. (1941). Determinants of apparent visual size with distance variant. *AJP, 54,* 21–37.

Ittelson, W. H. (1951a). Size as a cue to distance: Radial motion. *AJP, 64,* 188–192.

Ittelson, W. H. (1951b). The constancies in perceptual theory. *PR, 58,* 285–294.

Ittelson, W. H. (1952). *The Ames demonstrations in perception.* Princeton, NJ: Princeton University Press.

Ittelson, W. H. (1960). *Visual space perception.* New York: Springer.

Ittelson, W. H. (1968). *The Ames demonstrations in perception.* New York: Hafner Publishing Co.

Jansson, G., Burgström, S. S., & Epstein, W. (1994). *Perceiving events and objects.* Hillsdale, NJ: Erlbaum.

Jansson, G., & Johansson, G. (1973). Visual perception of bending motion. *Perception, 2,* 321–326.

Jansson, G., & Runeson, S. (1977). Perceived bending motion from a quadrangle changing form. *Perception, 6,* 595–600.

Johansson, G. (1950). *Configurations in event perception.* Uppsala, Sweden: Almqvist & Wiksells.

Johansson, G. (1958). Rigidity, stability, and motion in space perception. *Acta Psychologica, 14,* 359–370.

Johansson, G. (1964). Perception of motion and changing form. *Scandinavian Journal of Psychology, 5,* 181–208.

Johansson, G. (1970). On theories for visual space perception. A letter to Gibson. *Scandinavian Journal of Psychology, 11,* 67–74.

Johansson, G. (1973). Visual perception of biological motion and a model for its analysis. *P&P, 14,* 201–211.

Johansson, G. (1974a). Projective transformations as determining visual space perception. In R. B. MacLeod & H. L. Pick, Jr. (Eds.), *Perception: Essays in honor of James J. Gibson* (pp. 111–135). Ithaca, NY: Cornell University Press.

Johansson, G. (1974b). Vector analysis in visual perception of rolling motion: A quantitative approach. *Psychologiche Forschung, 36,* 311–319.

Johansson, G. (1977). Spatial constancy and motion in visual perception. In W. Epstein (Ed.), *Stability and constancy in visual perception: Mechanisms and processes* (pp. 375–419). New York: Wiley.

Johansson, G. (1978a). About the geometry underlying spontaneous visual decoding of the optical message. In E. L. J. Leeuwenberg & H. F. J. Buffart (Eds.), *Formal theories of visual perception* (pp. 265–276). New York: Wiley.

Johansson, G. (1978b). Visual event perception. In R. Held, H. W. Leibowitz, & H. L. Teuber (Eds.), *Handbook of sensory physiology, Vol. 8: Perception,* (pp. 675–711). New York: Springer.

Johansson, G. & Jansson, G. (1968). Perceived rotary motion from changes in a straight line. *P&P, 4,* 165–170.

Johansson, G., von Hofsten, C., & Jansson, G. (1980). Event perception. *Annual Review of Psychology, 31,* 27–63.

Julesz, B. (1960). Binocular depth perception of computer generated patterns. *Bell System Technical Journal, 39,* 1125–1162.

Julesz, B. (1971). *Foundations of cyclopean perception.* Chicago: University of Chicago Press.

Julesz, B. (1986). Stereoscopic vision. *VR, 26,* 1601–1612.

Kaiser, M. K., & Mowafy, L. (1993). Optical specification of time-to-passage: Observer's sensitivity to global tau. *JEP:HP&P, 19,* 1028–1040.

Kanizsa, G. (1955). Margini quasi-percettivi in campi con stimolazione omogenea. *Rivista di Psicologia, 49,* 7–30. [Also published as Quasiperceptual margins in homogeneously stimulated fields, trans. W. Gerbini, in S. Petry & G. E. Meyer (Eds.), *The perception of illusory contours* (pp. 40–49). New York: Springer-Verlag, 1987.]

Kaufman, L., & Rock, I. (1962). The moon illusion, I. *Science, 136,* 953–961.

Kaufman, L., & Rock, I. (1989). The moon illusion thirty years later. In M. Hershenson (Ed.), *The moon illusion* (pp. 193–234). Hillsdale, NJ: Erlbaum.

Kertesz, A. E. (1991). Cyclofusion. In D. Regan (Ed.), *Vision and visual dysfunction, Vol. 9: Binocular vision* (pp. 111–120). Boca Raton, FL: CRC Press.

Kilpatrick, F. R., & Ittelson, W. H. (1953). The size-distance invariance hypothesis. *PR, 60,* 223–231.

King, W. L., & Gruber, H. E. (1962). Moon illusion and Emmert's law. *Science, 135,* 1125–1126.

Kleffner, D. A. & Ramachandran, V. S. (1992). On the perception of shape from shading. *P&P, 52,* 18–36.

Koenderink, J. J. (1985). Space, form, and optical deformations. In D. A. Ingle, M. Jeannerod, & D. N. Lee, (Eds.), *Brain mechanisms and spatial vision* (pp. 31–58). Dordrecht, The Netherlands: Martinus Nijhoff.

Koenderink, J. J. (1986). Optic flow. *VR, 26,* 161–180.

Koenderink, J. J., & van Doorn, A. J. (1975). Invariant properties of the motion parallax field due to the motion of rigid bodies relative to the observer. *Optica Acta, 22,* 773–791.

Koenderink, J. J., & van Doorn, A. J. (1976). Local structure of movement parallax of a plane. *JOSA, 66,* 717–723.

Koenderink, J. J., & van Doorn, A. J. (1981). Exterospecific component of the motion parallax field. *JOSA, 71,* 953–957.

Koenderink, J. J., van Doorn, A. J., Christou, C., & Lappin, J. S. (1996). Perturbation study of shading in pictures. *Perception, 25,* 1009-1026.

Koffka, K. (1935). *Principles of Gestalt psychology.* New York: Harcourt Brace Jovanovich.

Köhler, W. (1929). *Gestalt psychology.* New York: Liveright.

Kolers, P. A. (1972). *Aspects of motion perception.* New York: Pergamon Press.

Lawson, R. B., & Gulick, W. L. (1967). Stereopsis and anomalous contours. *VR, 7,* 271–297.

Lee, D. N. (1974). Visual information during locomotion. In R. B. MacLeod & H. Pick (Eds.), *Perception: Essays in honor of James Gibson* (pp. 250–267). Ithaca, NY: Cornell University Press.

Lee, D. N. (1976). A theory of visual control of braking based on information about time-to-collision. *Perception, 5,* 437–459.

Lee, D. N. (1980). The optic flow field: The foundation of vision. *Philosophical Transactions of the Royal Society, London (B), 290,* 169–179.

Lee, D. N., & Aronson, E. (1974). Visual proprioceptive control of standing in human infants. *P&P, 15,* 529–532.

Lee, D. N., & Lishman, J. R. (1975). Visual proprioceptive control of stance. *Journal of Human Movement Studies, 1,* 87–95.

Lee, D. N., & Young, D. S. (1985). Visual timing of interceptive action. In D. Ingle, M. Jeannerod, & D. N. Lee (Eds.), *Brain mechanisms and spatial vision* (pp. 1–30). Dordrecht, The Netherlands: Martinus Nijhoff.

Leibowitz, H. W. (1974). Multiple mechanisms of size perception and size constancy. *Hiroshima Forum for Psychology, 1,* 47–53.

Leibowitz, H. W., & Harvey, L. O., Jr. (1967). Size matching as a function of instructions in a naturalistic environment. *JEP, 74,* 378–382.

Leibowitz, H. W., & Harvey, L. O., Jr. (1969). Effects of instructions, environment, and type of test object on matched size. *JEP, 81,* 36-43.

Leibowitz, H. W., Hennessy, R. T., & Owens, D. A. (1975). The intermediate resting position of accommodation and some implications for space perception. *Psychologia, 18,* 162–170.

Leibowitz, H. W., & Moore, D. (1966). Role of changes in accommodation and convergence in the perception of size. *JOSA, 56,* 1120–1123.

Leibowitz, H. W., & Owens, D. A. (1978). New evidence for the intermediate position of relaxed accommodation. *Documenta Ophthalmological, 46,* 133–147.

Leibowitz, H. W., Shiina, K., & Hennessy, R. T. (1972). Oculomotor adjustments and size constancy. *P&P, 12,* 497–500.

Lesher, G. W. (1995). Illusory contours: Toward a neurally based perceptual theory. *Psychonomic Bulletin & Review, 2,* 279–321.

Lettvin, J. Y., Maturana, H. R., McCulloch, W. S., & Pitts, W. H. (1959). What the frog's eye tells the frog's brain. *Proceedings of the IRE, 47,* 1940–1951.

Lettvin, J. Y., Maturana, H. R., Pitts, W. H., & McCulloch, W. S. (1961). Two remarks on the visual system of the frog. In W. S. Rosenblith (Ed.) *Sensory communication* (pp. 757–776). Cambridge, MA: MIT Press.

Levelt, W. J. M. (1968). *On binocular rivalry.* The Hague: Mouton.

Levin, C. A., & Haber, R. N. (1993). Visual angle as a determinant of perceived interobject distance. *P&P, 54,* 250–259.

Lichten, W., & Lurie, S. (1950). A new technique for the study of perceived size. *AJP, 63,* 280–282.

Lishman, J. R., & Lee, D. N. (1973). The autonomy of visual kinaesthesis. *Perception, 2,* 287–294.

Longuet-Higgins, H. C., & Prazdny, K. (1980). The interpretation of a moving retinal image. *Proceedings of the Royal Society of London, 208,* 385–397.

Lu, Z.-L., & Sperling, G. (1995). The functional architecture of human visual motion perception. *VR, 35,* 2697–2722.

Lu, Z.-L., & Sperling, G. (1996). Three systems for visual motion perception. *Current Directions in Psychological Science, 5,* 44–53.

Mack, A., Heuer, F., Fendrich, R., Vilardi, K., & Chambers, D. (1985). Induced motion and oculomotor capture. *JEP:HP&P, 11,* 329–345.

MacKay, D. M. (1973). Visual stability and voluntary eye movements. In R. Jung (Ed.), *Central processing of visual information.* New York: Springer.

Marr, D. & Poggio, T. (1976). Cooperative computation of stereo disparity. *Science, 194,* 283–287.

Massaro, D. W. (1973). The perception of rotated shapes: A process analysis of shape constancy. *P&P, 13,* 413–422.

McCready, D. (1965). Size-distance perception and accommodation-convergence micropsia: a critique. *VR, 5,* 189–206.

McCready, D. (1985). On size, distance, and visual angle perception. *P&P, 37,* 323–334.

McCready, D. (1986). Moon illusions redescribed. *P&P, 39,* 64–72.

Mitchison, G. J., & McKee, S. P. (1985). Interpolation in stereoscopic matching. *Nature, 315,* 402–404.

Mitchison, G. J., & McKee, S. P. (1987a). The resolution of ambiguous stereoscopic matches by interpolation. *VR, 27,* 285–294.

Mitchison, G. J., & McKee, S. P. (1987b). Interpolation and the detection of fine structure in stereoscopic matching. *VR, 27,* 295–302.

Morgan, M. J. (1991). Hyperacuity. In D. Regan (Ed.), *Vision and visual dysfunction, Vol. 10: Spatial vision* (pp. 88–113). Boca Raton, FL: CRC Press.

Musatti, C. L. (1924). Sui fenomeni stereocinetici. *Archivio Italiano de Psicologia, 3,* 105–120.

Myers, A. K. (1980). Quantitative indices of perceptual constancy. *PB, 88,* 451–457.

Nakayama, K. (1985). Extraction of higher order derivatives of the optical velocity vector field: Limitations imposed by biological hardware. In D. A. Ingle, M. Jeannerod, & D. N. Lee, (Eds.), *Brain mechanisms and spatial vision* (pp. 59–72). Dordrecht, The Netherlands: Martinus Nijhoff.

Nakayama, K., & Silverman, G. H. (1985). Sensitivity to shearing and compressive motion in random dots. *Perception, 14,* 225–238.

Norman, J. F. & Todd, J. T. (1994). The perception of rigid motion in depth from the optical deformations of shadows and occlusion boundaries. *JEP:HP&P, 29,* 343–356.

Ogle, K. N. (1950/1964). *Researches in binocular vision.* New York: Hafner.

Ogle, K. N. (1962a). Spatial localization according to direction. In H. Davson (Ed.), *The eye. Vol. 4: Visual optics and the optical space sense* (pp. 219–245). New York: Academic Press

Ogle, K. N. (1962b). Spatial localization through binocular vision. In H. Davson (Ed.), *The eye. Vol. 4: Visual optics and the optical space sense* (pp. 271–324). New York: Academic Press.

Ogle, K. N. (1962c). Special topics in binocular spatial localization. In H. Davson (Ed.), *The eye. Vol. 4: Visual optics and the optical space sense* (pp. 343–407). New York: Academic Press.

Ogle, K. N. (1962d). The problem of the horopter. In H. Davson (Ed.), *The eye. Vol. 4: Visual optics and the optical space sense* (pp. 325–348). New York: Academic Press.

Ono, H. (1979). Axiomatic summary and deduction from Hering's principles of visual direction. *P&P, 25,* 473–477.

Ono, H. (1981). On Wells's (1792) law of visual direction. *P&P, 30,* 403–406.

Ono, H. (1991). Binocular visual directions of an object when seen as single or double. In D. Regan (Ed.), *Vision and visual dysfunction, Vol. 9: Binocular vision* (pp. 1–17). Boca Raton, FL: CRC Press.

Ono, H. & Barbieto, R. (1982). The cyclopean eye vs. the sighting-dominant eye as the center of visual direction. *P&P, 32,* 201–210.

Ono, H., & Comerford, T. (1977). Stereoscopic depth constancy. In W. Epstein (Ed.), *Stability and constancy in visual perception: Mechanisms and processes* (pp. 91–128). New York: Wiley.

Ono, H., Rogers, B. J., Ohmi, M., & Ono, M. E. (1988). Dynamic occlusion and motion parallax in depth perception. *Perception, 17,* 255–266.

Ono, M. E., Rivest, J., & Ono, H. (1986). Depth perception as a function of motion parallax and absolute-distance information. *JEP:HP&P, 12,* 331-337.

O'Shea, R. P., Blackburn, S. G., & Ono, H. (1994). Contrast as a depth cue. *VR, 34,* 1595–1604.

Owens, D. A., & Leibowitz, H. W. (1983). Perceptual and motor consequences of tonic vergence. In C. M. Schor, & K. J. Ciuffreda (Eds.), *Vergence eye movements: Basic and clinical aspects* (pp. 25–74). Boston: Butterworth.

Oyama, T. (1977). Analysis of causal relations in the perceptual constancies. In W. Epstein (Ed.), *Stability and constancy in visual perception: Mechanisms and Processes* (pp. 183–216). New York: Wiley.

Panum, P.L. (1858). *Physiologische Untersuchengen über das Sehen mit zwei Augen.* Kiel: Schwering.

Pastore, N. (1971). *Selective history of theories of visual perception: 1650–1950.* New York: Oxford University Press.

Pentland, A. P. (1987). A new sense for depth of field. *IEEE Transactions on Pattern Analysis and Machine Intelligence, 9,* 523–531.

Pizlo, Z. (1994). A theory of shape constancy based on perspective invariants. *VR, 34,* 1637–1658.

Plug, C., & Ross, H. E. (1989). Historical review. In M. Hershenson (Ed.), *The moon illusion* (pp. 5–27). Hillsdale, NJ: Erlbaum.

Pollick, F. E., Watanabe, H., & Kawato, M. (1996). Perception of local orientation from shaded images. *P&P, 58,* 762–780.

Porac, C., & Coren, S. (1976). The dominant eye. *PB, 83,* 880–897.

Porac, C., & Coren, S. (1986). Sighting dominance and egocentric localization. *VR, 26,* 1709-1713.

Post, R. B., & Leibowitz, H. W. (1985). A revised analysis of the role of efference in motion perception. *Perception, 14,* 631–643.

Predebon, J. (1991). Spatial judgments of exocentric extents in an open-field situation: Familiar versus unfamiliar size. *P&P, 50,* 361–366.

Proffitt, D. R., Rock, I., Hecht, H., & Schubert, J. (1992). The stereokinetic effect and its relations to the kinetic depth effect. *JEP:HP&P, 18,* 3–21.

Purghé, F., & Coren, S. (1992). Subjective contours 1900–1990: Research trends and bibliography. *P&P, 51,* 291–304.

Ramachandran, V. S. (1988). Perception of shape from shading. *Nature, 331,* 163–166.

Regan, D. (1986a). Form from motion parallax and form from luminance contrast: vernier discrimination. *Spatial Vision, 1,* 305–318.

Regan, D. (1986b). Visual processing of four kinds of relative motion. *VR, 26,* 127–145.

Regan, D. (1991). Depth from motion and motion-in-depth. In D. Regan (Ed.), *Vision and visual dysfunction, Vol. 9: Binocular vision* (pp. 137–169). Boca Raton, FL: CRC Press.

Regan, D., & Beverley, K. I. (1978a). Illusory motion in depth: aftereffect of adaptation to changing size. *VR, 18,* 209–212.

Regan, D., & Beverley, K. I. (1978b). Looming detectors in the human visual pathway. *VR, 18,* 415–421.

Regan, D., & Beverley, K. I. (1979). Visually guided locomotion: psychophysical evidence for a neural mechanism sensitive to flow patterns. *Science, 205,* 311–313.

Regan, D., & Beverley, K. I. (1980). Visual response to changing size and to sideways motion for different directions of motion in depth. Linearization of visual responses. *JOSA, 70,* 1289–1296.

Regan, D., & Beverley, K. I. (1982). How do we avoid confounding the direction we are looking with the the direction we are moving. *Science, 215,* 194–196.

Regan, D., & Beverley, K. I. (1983). Visual fields for frontal plane motion and for changing size. *VR 23,* 673–676.

Regan, D. & Beverley, K. I. (1985). Visual response to vorticity and the neural analysis of optic flow. *JOSA, 2,* 280–283.

Reichardt, W. (1957). Autokorrelationsauswertung als Funktionsprinzip des Zentralnervensystems. *Zeitschrift Naturforschung, 12b,* 447–457.

Reichardt, W. (1961). Autocorrelation, a principle for the evaluation of sensory information by the central nervous system. In W. A. Rosenblith (Ed.), *Sensory Communication* (pp. 303–317). New York: Wiley.

Restle, F. (1982). Coding theory as an integration of Gestalt psychology and information processing theory. In J. Beck (Ed.), *Organization and representation in perception* (pp. 31–56). Hillsdale, NJ: Erlbaum.

Richards, W. (1975). Visual space perception. In E. C. Carterette, & M. P. Friedman (Eds.), *Handbook of perception, Vol. V: Seeing* (pp. 351–386). New York: Academic Press.

Richards, W., & Kaye, M. G. (1974). Local versus global stereopsis: two mechanisms? *VR, 14,* 1345–1347.

Rock, I. (1975). *An introduction to perception.* New York: Macmillan.

Rock, I. (1977). In defense of unconscious inference. In W. Epstein, (Ed.), *Stability and constancy in visual perception: Mechanisms and processes* (pp. 321–373). New York: Wiley.

Rock, I. (1983). *The logic of perception.* Cambridge, MA: MIT Press.

Rock, I., & Ebenholtz, S. (1959). The relational determination of perceived size. *PR, 66,* 387–401.

Rock, I., & Ebenholtz, S. (1962). Stroboscopic movement based on change of phenomenal rather than visual location. *AJP, 75,* 193–207.

Rock I., & Kaufman, L. (1962). The moon illusion, II. *Science, 136,* 1023–1031.

Rock, I., & McDermott, W. (1964). The perception of visual angle. *Acta Psychologica, 22,* 119–134.

Rock, I., Shallo, J., & Schwartz, F. (1978). Pictorial depth and related constancy effects as a function of recognition. *Perception, 7,* 3–19.

Rock, I., & Smith, D. (1981). Alternative solutions to kinetic stimulus transformations. *JEP:HP&P, 7,* 19–29.

Rogers, B., & Graham, M. (1979). Motion parallax as an independent cue for depth perception. *Perception, 8,* 125–134.

Rogers, B., & Graham, M. (1982). Similarities between motion parallax and stereopsis in human depth perception. *VR, 22,* 261–270.

Rogers, B., & Graham, M. (1985). Motion parallax and the perception of three-dimensional surfaces. In D. A. Ingle, M. Jeannerod, & D. N. Lee, (Eds.) *Brain mechanisms and spatial vision* (pp. 95–111). Dordrecht, The Netherlands: Martinus Nijhoff.

Roscoe, S. N. (1979). When day is done and shadows fall, we miss the airport most of all. *Human Factors, 21,* 721–731.

Roscoe, S. N. (1989). The zoom-lens hypothesis. In M. Hershenson, (Ed.), *The moon illusion* (pp. 59–121). Hillsdale, NJ: Erlbaum.

Rosinski, R. R., & Levine, N. P. (1976). Texture gradient effectiveness in the perception of surface slant. *Journal of Experimental Child Psychology, 22,* 261–271.

Runeson, S. (1988). The distorted room illusion, equivalent configurations, and the specificity of static optic arrays. *JEP:HP&P, 14,* 295–304.

Santen, J. P. H. van, & Sperling, G. (1984). Temporal covariance model of human motion perception. *JOSA, 1,* 451–473.

Schiff, W. (1965). Perception of impending collision: A study of visually directed avoidant behavior. *Psychological Monographs, 79,* Whole No. 604.

Schor, C. M. (1983). Fixation disparity and vergence adaptation. In C. M. Schor & K. J. Ciuffreda (Eds.), *Vergence eye movements: Basic and clinical aspects* (pp. 465–516). Boston: Butterworths.

Schor, C. M., Heckmann, T. & Tyler, C. W. (1989). Binocular fusion limits are independent of contrast, luminance gradient and component phases. *VR, 29,* 821–836.

Schor, C. M., & Tyler, C. W. (1981). Spatio-temporal properties of Panum's fusional area. *VR, 21,* 683–692.

Schor, C. M., Wood, I. & Ogawa, J. (1984). Binocular sensory fusion is limited by spatial resolution. *VR, 24,* 661–665.

Schumer, R. A. (1979). *Mechanisms in human stereopsis.* Thesis, Stanford University. Cited in Tyler (1991b).

Schur, E. (1925). Mondtäuschung und Sehgrössen konstanz. *Psychologische Forschung, 7,* 44–80.

Sedgwick, H. A. (1986). Space perception. In K. R. Boff, L. Kaufman, & J. P. Thomas (Eds.), *Handbook of perception and performance, Vol. I: Sensory processes (chapter 21).* New York: Wiley.

Sekuler, R. (1975). Visual motion perception. In E. C. Carterette, & M. P. Friedman (Eds.), *Handbook of perception, Vol. V: Seeing* (pp. 387–430). New York: Academic Press.

Sekuler, R. (1996). Motion perception: A modern view of Wertheimer's 1912 monograph. *Perception*, 25, 1243-1258.

Sekuler, R., Pantle, A., & Levinson, E. (1978). Physiological basis for motion perception. In R. Held, H. W. Leibowitz, & H.-L. Teuber (Eds.), *Handbook of sensory physiology, VIII,: Perception.* Berlin: Springer Verlag.

Sheedy, J. E. & Fry, G. A. (1979). The perceived direction of the binocular image. *VR*, 19, 201-211.

Shepard, R. N., & Judd, S. A. (1976). Perceptual illusion of rotation of three-dimensional objects. *Science*, 191, 952–954.

Shimojo, S., & Nakajima, Y. (1981). Adaptation to the reversal of binocular depth cues: effects of wearing left-right reversing spectacles on stereoscopic depth perception. *Perception*, 10, 391–402.

Solhkhah, N., & Orbach, J. (1969). Determinants of the magnitude of the moon illusion. *Perceptual and Motor Skills*, 29, 87–98.

Swanston, M. T., & Gogel, W. C. (1986). Perceived size and motion in depth from optical expansion. *P&P*, 39, 309–326.

Tanaka, K., & Saito, H. (1989). Analysis of motion of the visual field by direction, expansion/contraction and rotation cells clustered in the dorsal part of the medial superior temporal area of the Macaque monkey. *Journal of Neurophysiology*, 62, 626–641.

Taylor, D. W., & Boring, E. G. (1942). The moon illusion as a function of binocular regard. *AJP*, 55, 189–201.

Teghtsoonian, M. (1974). The doubtful phenomenon of over-constancy. In H. R. Moskowitz, B. Scharf, & J. C. Stevens (Eds.), *Sensation and measurement.* Dordrecht, The Netherlands: Reidel.

Thouless, R. H. (1931). Phenomenal regression to the real object: I. *British Journal of Psychology*, 21, 339–359.

Todd, J. T. (1982). Visual information about rigid and nonrigid motion: A geometric analysis. *JEP:HP&P*, 8, 238–252.

Todd, J. T. (1984). The perception of three-dimensional structure from rigid and nonrigid motion. *P&P*, 36, 97–103.

Todd, J. (1985). The analysis of three-dimensional structure from moving images. In D. A. Ingle, M. Jeannerod, & D. N. Lee, (Eds.), *Brain mechanisms and spatial vision* (pp. 73–93). Dordrecht, The Netherlands: Martinus Nijhoff.

Toye, R. C. (1986). The effect of viewing position on the perceived layout of space. *P&P*, 40, 85-92.

Tresilian, J. R. (1991). Empirical and theoretical issues in the perception of time to contact. *JEP:HP&P*, 17, 865–876.

Tyler, C. W. (1973). Stereoscopic vision: Cortical limitations and a disparity scaling effect. *Science*, 181, 276–278.

Tyler, C. W. (1983). Sensory processing of binocular disparity. In C. M. Schor & K. J. Ciuffreda (Eds.), *Vergence eye movements: Basic and clinical aspect* (pp. 199–295). London: Butterworths.

Tyler, C. W. (1991a). Cyclopean vision. In D. Regan (Ed.), *Vision and visual dysfunction, Vol. 9: Binocular vision* (pp. 38–74). Boca Raton, FL: CRC Press.

Tyler, C. W. (1991b). The horopter and binocular fusion. In D. Regan (Ed.), *Vision and visual dysfunction, Vol. 9: Binocular vision* (pp. 19-37). Boca Raton, FL: CRC Press.

Tyler, C. W., & Chang, J. J. (1977). Visual echoes: the perception of repetition in quasi-random patterns. *VR, 17,* 109–116.

Tyler, C. W., & Julesz, B. (1976). The neural transfer characteristic (neurontropy) for binocular stochastic stimulation. *Biological Cybernetics, 23,* 33–37.

Tynan, P., & Sekuler, R. (1975). Moving visual phantoms: A new contour completion effect. *Science, 188,* 951–952.

Ullman, S. (1979a). *The interpretation of visual motion.* Cambridge, MA: MIT Press.

Ullman, S. (1979b). The interpretation of structure from motion. *Proceedings of the Royal Society, London, B, 203,* 405–426.

Van den Berg, A. V. (1992). Robustness of perception of heading from optic flow. *VR, 32,* 1285–1296.

von Holst, E. (1954). Relations between the central nervous system and the peripheral organs. *British Journal of Animal Behaviour, 2,* 89–94.

Vickers, D. (1971). Perceptual economy and the impression of depth. *P&P, 10,* 23–27.

Wagner, M. (1985). The metric of visual space. *P&P, 38,* 483–495.

Wallach, H. (1935). Über visuall wahrgenommene Bewegungsrichtung. *Psychologische Forschung, 20,* 325–380.

Wallach, H. (1976). *On perception.* New York: Quadrangle.

Wallach, H. (1984). Learning in space perception. In L. Spillman & B. R. Wooten (Eds.), *Sensory experience, adaptation, and perception* (pp. 353–363). Hillsdale, NJ: Erlbaum.

Wallach, H., & Berson, E. (1989). Measurements of the illusion. In M. Hershenson (Ed.), *The moon illusion* (pp. 287–297). Hillsdale, NJ: Erlbaum.

Wallach, H., & Floor, L. (1971). The use of size matching to demonstrate the effectiveness of accommodation and convergence as cues for distance. *P&P, 10,* 423–428.

Wallach, H., & Frey, K. J. (1972). Adaptation in distance perception based on oculomotor cues. *P&P, 11,* 77–83.

Wallach, H., & O'Connell, D. N. (1953). The kinetic depth effect. *JEP, 45,* 205–217.

Wallach, H., Weisz, A., & Adams, P. A. (1956). Circles and derived figures in rotation. *AJP, 69,* 48–59.

Wallach, H., & Zuckerman, C. (1963). The constancy of stereoscopic depth. *AJP, 76,* 404–412.

Warren, W. II. Jr., Morris, M. W., & Kalish, M. (1988). Perception of translational heading from optical flow. *JEP:HP&P, 14,* 646–660.

Weinshall, D., & Malik, J. (1994). Review of computational models of stereopsis. In T. V. Papathomas, C. Chubb, A.M Gorea, & E. Kowler (Eds.), *Early vision and beyond* (pp. 33–41). Cambridge, MA: MIT Press.

Weintraub, D. J., & Gardner, G. T. (1970). Emmert's law: Size constancy versus optical geometry. *AJP. 83,* 40–54.

Weisstein, N., & Maguire, W. (1978). Computing the next step: Psychophysical measures of representation and interpretation. In A. L. Hanson & E. M. Riseman (Eds.), *Computer vision systems.* New York: Academic Press.

Weisstein, N., Maguire, W., & Berbaum, K. (1977). A phantom-motion aftereffect. *Science, 189,* 955-958.

Weisstein, N., Maguire, W., & Williams, M. C. (1982). The effect of perceived depth on phantoms and the phantom motion aftereffect. In J. Beck (Ed.), *Organization and representation in perception* (pp. 235–249). Hillsdale, NJ: Erlbaum.

Wertheimer, M. (1912). Experimentelle Studien über das Sehen von Bewegung. *Zeitschrift für Psychologie, 61,* 161–265.

Wertheimer, M. (1923/1937). Laws of organization in perceptual forms. In W. D. Ellis (Ed.), *A source-book in Gestalt psychology.* London: Routledge & Kegan Paul (Original in German).

Westheimer, G. (1979a). Cooperative neural processes involved in stereoscopic acuity. *Experimental Brain Research, 36,* 585–597.

Westheimer, G. (1979b). The spatial sense of the eye. *Investigative Ophthalmology and Visual Science, 18,* 893–912.

Wheatstone, C. (1838). Contributions to the physiology of vision. Part the first. On some remarkable, and hitherto unobserved, phenomena of binocular vision. *Philosophical Transactions, Royal Society of London, 128,* 371–394.

Wiest, W. M., & Bell, B. (1985). Steven's exponent for psychophysical scaling of perceived, remembered, and inferred distance. *PB, 98,* 457–470.

Wilson, H. R. (1991). Psychophysical models of spatial vision and hyperacuity. In D. Regan (Ed.), *Vision and visual dysfunction, Vol. 10: Spatial vision* (pp. 64–86). Boca Raton, FL: CRC Press.

Zanforlin, M. (1988). The height of a stereokinetic cone: A quantitative determination of a 3-D effect from 2-D moving patterns without a "rigidity assumption." *Psychological Research, 50,* 162–172.

Name Index

Subject Index